Hidradenitis Suppurativa

Editor

GREGOR B.E. JEMEC

DERMATOLOGIC CLINICS

www.derm.theclinics.com

Consulting Editor
BRUCE H. THIERS

January 2016 • Volume 34 • Number 1

ELSEVIER

1600 John F. Kennedy Boulevard • Suite 1800 • Philadelphia, Pennsylvania, 19103-2899

http://www.theclinics.com

DERMATOLOGIC CLINICS Volume 34, Number 1
January 2016 ISSN 0733-8635, ISBN-13: 978-0-323-41449-4

Editor: Jessica McCool
Developmental Editor: Alison Swety

Dermatologic Clinics (ISSN 0733-8635) is published quarterly by Elsevier Inc., 360 Park Avenue South, New York, NY 10010-1710. Months of publication are January, April, July, and October. Business and editorial offices: 1600 John F. Kennedy Blvd., Suite 1800, Philadelphia, PA 19103-2899. Customer service office: 11830 Westline Drive, St. Louis, MO 63146. Periodicals postage paid at New York, NY, and additional mailing offices. Subscription prices are USD 370.00 per year for US individuals, USD 618.00 per year for US institutions, USD 425.00 per year for Canadian individuals, USD 754.00 per year for Canadian institutions, USD 495.00 per year for international individuals, USD 754.00 per year for international institutions, USD 100.00 per year for US students/residents, and USD 240.00 per year for Canadian and international students/residents. International air speed delivery is included in all *Clinics* subscription prices. All prices are subject to change without notice. **POSTMASTER:** Send address changes to *Dermatologic Clinics*, Elsevier Health Sciences Division, Subscription Customer Service, 3251 Riverport Lane, Maryland Heights, MO 63043. **Customer Service: 1-800-654-2452 (U.S. and Canada); 314-447-8871 (outside U.S. and Canada). Fax: 314-447-8029. E-mail: journalscustomerservice-usa@elsevier.com (for print support); journalsonlinesupport-usa@elsevier.com (for online support).**

Reprints. For copies of 100 or more, of articles in this publication, please contact the Commercial Reprints Department, Elsevier Inc., 360 Park Avenue South, New York, New York 10010-1710. Tel.: 212-633-3874; Fax: 212-633-3820; Email: reprints@elsevier.com.

The *Dermatologic Clinics* is covered in *MEDLINE/PubMed (Index Medicus), Current Contents/Clinical Medicine, Excerpta Medica, Chemical Abstracts,* and *ISI/BIOMED.*

Contributors

CONSULTING EDITOR

BRUCE H. THIERS, MD
Professor and Chairman, Department of Dermatology and Dermatologic Surgery, Medical University of South Carolina, Charleston, South Carolina

EDITOR

GREGOR B.E. JEMEC, MD, DMSc
Professor and Chairman, Department of Dermatology, Roskilde Hospital, Health Sciences Faculty, University of Copenhagen, Roskilde, Denmark

AUTHORS

VINCENZO BETTOLI, MD
Department of Clinical and Experimental Medicine, OU of Dermatology, Azienda Ospedaliera – University of Ferrara, Ferrara, Italy

ANDRZEJ BIENIEK, MD, PhD
Department of Dermatology, Wroclaw Medical University, University of Wrocław, Wrocław, Poland

JURR BOER, MD, PhD
Department of Dermatology, Deventer Hospital, Deventer, The Netherlands

CORRADO CAMPOCHIARO, MD
Unit of Medicine and Clinical Immunology, IRCCS San Raffaele Scientific Institute, Vita-Salute San Raffaele University, Milan, Italy

LORENZO DAGNA, MD, FACP, FEFIM (Hon)
Unit of Medicine and Clinical Immunology, IRCCS San Raffaele Scientific Institute, Vita-Salute San Raffaele University, Milan, Italy

INGE ELIZABETH DECKERS, MD
Department of Dermatology, Erasmus MC, University Medical Center Rotterdam, Rotterdam, The Netherlands

LENNART EMTESTAM, MD
Professor, Department of Dermatology and Venereology, Karolinska University Hospital, Stockholm, Sweden

WAYNE GULLIVER, BSc, MD, FRCPC, FACP
Faculty of Medicine, Memorial University of Newfoundland, St. John's, Newfoundland and Labrador, Canada

ILTEFAT HAMZAVI, MD
Senior Staff Physician, Department of Dermatology, Multicultural Dermatology Center, Henry Ford Hospital, Detroit, Michigan

BARBARA HORVÁTH, MD, PhD
Department of Dermatology, University Medical Center Groningen, University of Groningen, Groningen, The Netherlands

JOHN R. INGRAM, MA, MSc, DM, MRCP(Derm), FAcadMEd
Senior Lecturer and Consultant Dermatologist, Department of Dermatology and Wound Healing, University Hospital of Wales, Cardiff University, Cardiff, United Kingdom

INEKE JANSE, MD
Department of Dermatology, University Medical Center Groningen, University of Groningen, Groningen, The Netherlands

GREGOR B.E. JEMEC, MD, DMSc
Professor and Chairman, Department of Dermatology, Roskilde Hospital, Health Sciences Faculty, University of Copenhagen, Roskilde, Denmark

OLIVIER JOIN-LAMBERT, MD, PhD
Department of Microbiology, INSERM UMR 1151, Team 11 Necker Enfants-Malades Hospital, Paris, France

IOANNIS KARAGIANNIDIS, MD
Departments of Dermatology, Allergology, Venereology, and Immunology, Dessau Medical Center, Dessau, Germany

G. KELLY, MB, MRCPI
Department of Dermatology, St. Vincent's University Hospital, Dublin, Ireland

ALEXA BOER KIMBALL, MD, MPH
Department of Dermatology, Harvard Medical School, Boston, Massachusetts

JAN LAPINS, MD, DMSc
Department of Dermatology, Karolinska University Hospital, Stockholm, Sweden

ŁUKASZ MATUSIAK, MD, PhD
Department of Dermatology, Wroclaw Medical University, University of Wrocław, Wrocław, Poland

RACHEL J. McANDREW, MD
Department of Dermatology, Henry Ford Hospital, Detroit, Michigan

JAN R. MEKKES, MD, PhD
Department of Dermatology, Academic Medical Center, University of Amsterdam, Amsterdam, The Netherlands

IBEN MARIE MILLER, MD, PhD
Department of Dermatology, Roskilde Hospital, Roskilde, Denmark

AUDE NASSIF, MD
Medical Center, Institut Pasteur, Paris, France

MAIWAND NAZARY, MSc
Division of Pharmacology, Utrecht Institute for Pharmaceutical Sciences, University of Utrecht, Utrecht, The Netherlands

GEORGIOS NIKOLAKIS, MD, PhD
Departments of Dermatology, Allergology, Venereology, and Immunology, Dessau Medical Center, Dessau, Germany

ERROL P. PRENS, MD, PhD
Department of Dermatology, Erasmus University Medical Centre Rotterdam, Rotterdam, Netherlands

JEAN E. REVUZ, MD, PhD
Professor, Private Practice, Paris, France

PETER THEUT RIIS, MD
Department of Dermatology, Roskilde Hospital, Roskilde, Denmark

HANS CHRISTIAN RING, MD
Department of Dermatology, Roskilde Hospital, University of Copenhagen, Roskilde, Denmark

DITTE M. SAUNTE, MD, PhD
Department of Dermatology, Roskilde Hospital, Roskilde, Denmark

THRASIVOULOS TZELLOS, MD, MSc, PhD
Department of Dermatology, Faculty of Health Sciences, University Hospital of North Norway, Troms, Norway

HESSEL H. VAN DER ZEE, MD, PhD
Department of Dermatology, Erasmus Medical Center, Rotterdam, The Netherlands

DOMINIQUE C. VAN RAPPARD, MD
Department of Dermatology, Academic Medical Center, University of Amsterdam, Amsterdam, The Netherlands

XIMENA WORTSMAN, MD
Adjunct Associate Professor, Departments of Radiology and Dermatology, Institute for Diagnostic Imaging and Research of the Skin and Soft Tissues, Clinica Servet, Faculty of Medicine, University of Chile, Santiago, Chile

CHRISTOS C. ZOUBOULIS, MD, PhD
Departments of Dermatology, Allergology, Venereology, and Immunology, Dessau Medical Center, Dessau, Germany

Contents

Chinese patients had a severe disease phenotype, with involvement of nonflexural skin locations such as the back and chest. These findings have been replicated in European populations, but g-secretase mutations have been found only in a minority of patients with HS.

The Microbiology of Hidradenitis Suppurativa 29

Hans Christian Ring and Lennart Emtestam

Although the clinical presentation of Hidradenitis Suppurativa (HS) is strongly reminiscent of bacterial infection, the role of bacteria remains controversial. Studies have isolated an array of different bacterial specimens as well as biofilm formation in lesional HS skin. Consistent findings of Gram-positive cocci and -rods including *Staphylococus aureus*, *Coagulase-negative staphylococci* (CoNS) and *Corynebacterium species* (spp) in deep tissue samples have been demonstrated in HS. Although efficacy of antibiotics, i.e. rifampicin, clindamycin or tetracycline may support a microbial role in disease pathogenesis, the most often isolated bacterial specimens are commensal bacteria (CoNS).

The Role of Mechanical Stress in Hidradenitis Suppurativa 37

Jurr Boer, Maiwand Nazary, and Peter Theut Riis

Mechanical stress can act as a possible trigger in the development of hidradenitis suppurativa (HS). The mechanical stress has been supported by (1) the special biomechanical conditions in the typically topographic areas of HS; (2) the indirect proof of similar findings in associated follicular occlusion diseases such as acne mechanica and pilonidal sinus disease, and in limb amputees after expression of mechanical forces; (3) pathohistologic, ultrasonography, and immunologic findings; and (4) overweight patients seem to be most susceptible to the effects of mechanical stress.

Endocrinologic Aspects of Hidradenitis Suppurativa 45

Ioannis Karagiannidis, Georgios Nikolakis, and Christos C. Zouboulis

Hidradenitis suppurativa (HS) is a chronic inflammatory skin disorder of unknown etiology. The role of hormones in HS remains unclear, but the observation of premenstrual flares, female predominance, and improvement during pregnancy suggest a hormonal/metabolic background. The reported positive effects of antiandrogen therapy supports a possible role of androgens. The predominant onset of the disease years after puberty may indicate a metabolic disorder. Obesity contributes significantly to HS pathogenesis; diabetes, dyslipidemia, the metabolic syndrome, and polycystic ovarian syndrome are among the commonest comorbidities. More studies are required to clarify a potential hormonal dysregulation in HS.

Inflammatory Mechanisms in Hidradenitis Suppurativa 51

G. Kelly and Errol P. Prens

Hidradenitis suppurativa (HS) is a chronic relapsing disease of follicular occlusion that causes immense clinical and psychosocial morbidity when refractory to treatment. HS is no longer considered a disease of primary infectious etiology, although bacteria play a role. There is increasing evidence that HS is associated with immune dysregulation, based on its clinical association with other immune-mediated disorders, by its response to biologic therapy in the clinical arena, and from molecular research. This article summarizes what is known in relation to the inflammatory pathways in HS.

Imaging of Hidradenitis Suppurativa 59

Ximena Wortsman

 Videos of Power Doppler and gray scale ultrasound accompany this article

Hidradenitis suppurativa is a complex disease of chronic evolution and difficult management. Imaging, particularly color Doppler ultrasound, has demonstrated a wide range of subclinical anatomic abnormalities, allowing modification of the clinical assessment of severity of the disease and therefore management of patients. Sonography supports early and more precise diagnosis and staging by providing critical objective information in real time. The richness of these data can also support assessment of the pathogenesis of the disease, allow monitoring of patients, and contribute to clinical trials. MRI can support the diagnosis of extensive anogenital and deep lesions.

Randomized Controlled Trials for the Treatment of Hidradenitis Suppurativa 69

Dominique C. van Rappard, Jan R. Mekkes, and Thrasivoulos Tzellos

Hidradenitis suppurativa (HS) is a chronic, inflammatory, recurrent, debilitating skin disease. Several treatment modalities are available, but most of them lack high-quality evidence. A systematic search was performed to identify all randomized controlled trials for the treatment of HS in order to review and evaluate the evidence. Recommendations for future randomized controlled trials include using validated scores, inclusion of patient rated outcomes, and thorough report of side effects. Evidence for long-term treatment and benefit/risk ratio of available treatment modalities is needed in order to enhance evidence-based treatment in daily clinical practice. Combining surgery with antiinflammatory treatment warrants further investigation.

Antibiotic Treatment of Hidradenitis Suppurativa 81

Vincenzo Bettoli, Olivier Join-Lambert, and Aude Nassif

Although hidradenitis suppurativa (HS) is not primarily an infectious disease, antibiotics are widely used to treat HS. Recent microbiological data show that HS lesions are associated with pathogenic commensal bacteria that can cause soft tissue and skin infections. Analysis of the literature provides little information on the efficacy of antibiotics in HS but suggests a beneficial effect of certain antimicrobial treatments including remission, depending on the clinical severity of the disease. Prospective studies are needed to confirm and optimize the efficacy of AB in HS.

Medical Treatments of Hidradenitis Suppurativa: More Options, Less Evidence 91

Hessel H. van der Zee and Wayne Gulliver

Hidradenitis suppurativa is a common debilitating skin disease that has been neglected by science.There is a need for effective treatment. We are still at the beginning of improving care for these patients as demonstrated by the low levels of evidence. The following treatments have a category of evidence of III and a strength of recommendation of C. Acitretin, metformin and zinc gluconate. The following treatments have a category of evidence of IV and a strength of recommendation of D. Ustekinumab, steroids (intralesional/systemic), dapsone, cyclosporine,

DERMATOLOGIC CLINICS

FORTHCOMING ISSUES

April 2016
Advances in Acne Management
James Q. Del Rosso and Joshua A. Zeichner, *Editors*

July 2016
Practice Gaps in Dermatology
Murad Alam, *Editor*

October 2016
Confocal Microscopy
Jane M. Grant-Kels, Giovanni Pellacani, and Caterina Longo, *Editors*

RECENT ISSUES

October 2015
Cutaneous Lymphoma
Elise A. Olsen, *Editor*

July 2015
Granulomatous Disorders of Adult Skin
Joseph C. English III, *Editor*

April 2015
Nail Disorders: Practical Tips for Diagnosis and Treatment
Antonella Tosti, *Editor*

ISSUE OF RELATED INTEREST

Primary Care: Clinics in Office Practice, December 2015 (Vol. 42, No. 4)
Primary Care Dermatology
George G.A. Pujalte, *Editor*
Available at: http://www.primarycare.theclinics.com/

THE CLINICS ARE AVAILABLE ONLINE!
Access your subscription at:
www.theclinics.com

Letter to the Editor

BRAF Mutations in Erdheim-Chester Disease

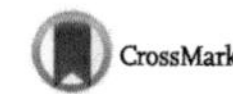

Erdheim-Chester disease (ECD) is a xanthogranulomatous disease with variable manifestations[1,2] that can also severely involve the orbit. In their recent article, "Adult orbital xanthogranulomatous disease: a review with emphasis on etiology, systemic associations, diagnostic tools, and treatment," published in *Dermatologic Clinics*, Justin Kerstetter and Jun Wang portray a global picture of the various conditions that may present as orbital xanthogranulomatous disease, with a particular focus on systemic diseases.[3] Recent and crucial discoveries in the field of ECD are not included in their review and should be addressed. First of all, the BRAF mutation V600E has been identified by several groups in most of the patients with ECD.[4,5] BRAF is a serine/threonine protein kinase, with a crucial role in the regulation of cell proliferation and survival, as it contributes to the RAS-RAF-MEK-ERK protein kinase pathway.[6] More recently, other more sporadic mutations in genes associated with a chronic activation of this pathway have been described in ECD patients.[7] The oncogenic activation of the MAP kinase pathway has also been associated with oncogene-induced senescence, a protective mechanism against oncogenic events, whose activation leads to cell-cycle arrest and induction of pro-inflammatory molecules, events that are characteristically seen in ECD.[8] These important insights in the pathogenesis of ECD have fundamental therapeutic implications, since BRAFV600E is a drug-targetable mutation. It has indeed been shown that ECD patients treated with vemurafenib, a selective BRAF V600E inhibitor, encounter a dramatic clinical and radiographic improvement.[9,10] These results have made vemurafenib one of the main cornerstones of the recently published guidelines on the management of ECD,[11] particularly when the disease is advanced, diffuse, or severe.[1,6,12,13]

Corrado Campochiaro, MD
Unit of Medicine and Clinical Immunology
IRCCS San Raffaele Scientific Institute
Vita-Salute San Raffaele University
Via Olgettina 60
20132 Milan, Italy

Lorenzo Dagna, MD, FACP, FEFIM (Hon)
Unit of Medicine and Clinical Immunology
IRCCS San Raffaele Scientific Institute
Vita-Salute San Raffaele University
Via Olgettina 60
20132 Milan, Italy

E-mail addresses:
corrado.campochiaro@hsr.it (C. Campochiaro)
lorenzo.dagna@unisr.it (L. Dagna)

REFERENCES

1. Cavalli G, Guglielmi B, Berti A, et al. The multifaceted clinical presentations and manifestations of Erdheim-Chester disease: comprehensive review of the literature and of 10 new cases. Ann Rheum Dis 2013;72:1691–5.
2. Cavalli G, Berti A, Campochiaro C, et al. Diagnosing Erdheim-Chester disease. Ann Rheum Dis 2013;72:e19.
3. Kerstetter J, Wang J. Adult orbital xanthogranulomatous disease. A review with emphasis on etiology, systemic associations, diagnostic tools, and treatment. Dermatol Clin 2015;33:457–63.
4. Haroche J, Charlotte F, Arnaud L, et al. High prevalence of BRAF V600E mutations in Erdheim-Chester disease but not in other non-Langerhans cell histiocytoses. Blood 2012;120:2700–3.
5. Cangi MG, Biavasco R, Cavalli G, et al. BRAFV600E-mutation is invariably present and associated to oncogene-induced senescence in Erdheim-Chester disease. Ann Rheum Dis 2015;74:1596–602.
6. Campochiaro C, Tomelleri A, Cavalli G, et al. Erdheim-Chester disease. Eur J Intern Med 2015;26:223–9.
7. Emile JF, Diamond EL, Hélias-Rodzewicz Z, et al. Recurrent RAS and PIK3CA mutations in Erdheim-Chester disease. Blood 2014;124:3016–9.
8. Cavalli G, Biavasco R, Borgiani B, et al. Oncogene-induced senescence as a new mechanism of disease: the paradigm of Erdheim-Chester disease. Front Immunol 2014;5:281.
9. Haroche J, Cohen-Aubart F, Emile JF, et al. Dramatic efficacy of vemurafenib in both multisystemic and refractory Erdheim-Chester disease and Langerhans cell histiocytosis harboring the BRAF V600E mutation. Blood 2013;121:1495–500.

Dermatol Clin 34 (2016) xi–xii
http://dx.doi.org/10.1016/j.det.2015.10.002

10. Haroche J, Cohen-Aubart F, Emile JF, et al. Reproducible and sustained efficacy of targeted therapy with vemurafenib in patients with BRAF(V600E)-mutated Erdheim-Chester disease. J Clin Oncol 2015;33:411–8.
11. Diamond EL, Dagna L, Hyman DM, et al. Consensus guidelines for the diagnosis and clinical management of Erdheim-Chester disease. Blood 2014;124:483–92.
12. Haroche J, Amoura Z, Trad SG, et al. Variability in the efficacy of interferon-alpha in Erdheim-Chester disease by patient and site of involvement: results in eight patients. Arthritis Rheum 2006;54:3330–6.
13. Berti A, Ferrarini M, Ferrero E, et al. Cardiovascular manifestations of Erdheim-Chester disease. Clin Exp Rheumatol 2015;33:S155–63.

Preface
The Secret Scourge

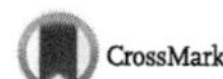

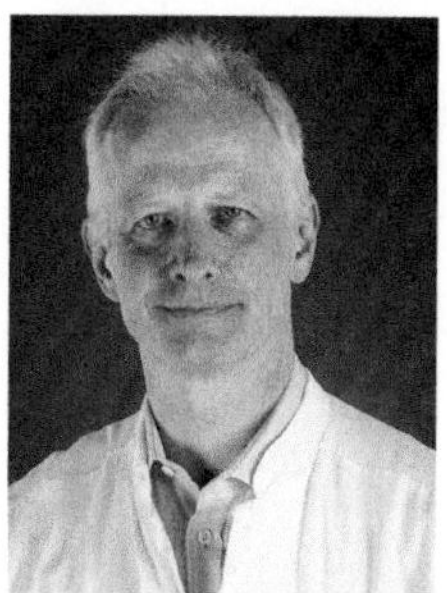

Gregor B.E. Jemec, MD, DMSc
Editor

Some diseases have a greater impact than others. Hidradenitis suppurativa (HS) is a high-impact disease, not only due to its signs and symptoms but also because of the psychosocial connotations of the predominant signs. Most patients primarily associate HS with its inflamed lesions, which they commonly describe as boils. Boils are a culturally laden concept that elicits associations to something unclean and contagious in most people, making HS a very stigmatizing disease. While it is therefore lucky that HS lesions usually remain hidden, other inherent features of HS contribute to the plight of patients. In particular, the risk of sudden malodourous discharge and pain burden the patients. The diagnosis of HS is furthermore associated with a significant delay, indicating that there is a substantial group of patients with an unmet need of both diagnosis and subsequent treatment globally.

The literature on HS is growing rapidly, and this issue of *Dermatologic Clinics* is therefore an important milestone. It brings together an eminent group of interested specialists with a long and proven history of expertise in the area of HS to provide the reader with both evidence and an updated expert appraisal. The authors cover many important aspects of HS, sometimes challenging our understanding of the pathogenesis of the disease, sometimes providing guidance to treatment and management of the many patients that are making their presence felt in clinics all over the world.

It is therefore my hope that this issue will help promote three important aspects of HS: one clinical, one academic, and one professional. First and foremost, it is intended to aid the many colleagues who are treating these patients all over the world in the practical management of the disease. Patients have an unmet need for diagnosis and treatment, which I hope this issue will help alleviate. Second, one may hope that the reviews of possible causes and pathogenesis may inspire more people to get involved in the exploration of this complex disease and strengthen the academic interest. Academic interest not only helps us meet current challenges but also provides a better understanding of the complex mechanisms that may also be involved in other diseases, providing new insights and more solutions in the future. Finally, this issue is a professional statement, reminding us all that skin diseases are not merely cosmetic problems.

I would like to thank the authors for their generous and enthusiastic contributions to this issue; may many patients derive benefit from these texts.

Gregor B.E. Jemec, MD, DMSc
Department of Dermatology
Roskilde Hospital
University of Copenhagen
Køgevej 7
DK-4000 Roskilde, Denmark

E-mail address:
gbj@regionsjaelland.dk

Dermatol Clin 34 (2016) xiii
http://dx.doi.org/10.1016/j.det.2015.10.001
0733-8635/16/$ – see front matter

Diagnosing Hidradenitis Suppurativa

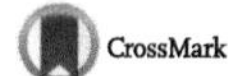

Jean E. Revuz, MD, PhD[a], Gregor B.E. Jemec, MD, DMSc[b,*]

KEYWORDS

- Hidradenitis suppurativa • Diagnostic criteria • Signs • Patient-reported outcome measures
- Quality of life • Comorbidity

KEY POINTS

- Hidradenitis suppurativa (HS) is a clinical diagnosis.
- Three diagnostic criteria must be met: (1) typical lesions, that is, deep-seated painful nodules; (2) typical location, that is, the disease must occur in 1 or more of the predilection areas, including axillae, inframammary and intermammary folds, groin, perineal region, or buttocks; and (3) typical evolution, that is, a chronic and/or recurrent disease.
- Recommended overall outcome measures include general patient-reported outcome measures such as patient-reported pain and itch scales, Dermatology Life Quality Index, and Skindex.
- HS is associated with significant comorbidities; in particular, metabolic syndrome and depression, which must be addressed in the evaluation of the patient.

Hidradenitis suppurativa (HS) is a clinically defined disease, with no pathognomonic tests. This is not unique among dermatologic diseases but this requires clearly stated criteria. It may contribute to the significant diagnostic and, consequently, therapeutic delay many patients experience.[1] In addition to diagnosis, research and patient management also benefit from standardized and validated outcome reporting. Although consensus has been reached on the diagnostic criteria, the outcomes reported still vary considerably. The explicit use of the definitions and outcome measures described in this article is recommended in future studies.

DIAGNOSIS

The diagnosis is given by the modified Dessau definition, describing diagnostic lesions, topography, and history of the disease.[2] Although the modified Dessau definition is usually straightforward, the terminology used to describe HS has not been consistent throughout the literature.[3]

Three criteria must be present:

1. Typical lesions, that is, deep-seated painful nodules. These are often described as blind boils in the early lesions because they do not have a purulent point, presumably due to their deeper location in the dermis. Other lesions that are commonly described are: abscesses; bridged scars; draining sinus (inflamed tunnels); and postinflammatory, open, tombstone double-ended comedones (pseudocomedones). Patients often indiscriminately describe the lesions as boils. Usually, multiple elements are present that facilitate the diagnosis. It is, however, important to avoid confusion with nondiagnostic elements, such as simple folliculitis, when making the diagnosis.

Disclosures: Neither author has any relevant conflict of interest to disclose. G.B.E. Jemec: Unrestricted grants from Leo Pharma and Abbvie; investigator for Abbvie, Novartis, Regeneron; advisory boards or consultant for Abbvie, Leo pharma, Novaris, MSD, Janssen-Cilag; speaker for Abbvie, Galderma, MSD.

[a] Private Practice, 11 chaussée de la Muette, Paris 75016, France; [b] Department of Dermatology, Roskilde Hospital, Health Sciences Faculty, University of Copenhagen, Køgevej 7-13, Roskilde DK-4000, Denmark
* Corresponding author.
E-mail address: gbj@regionsjaelland.dk

Dermatol Clin 34 (2016) 1–5
http://dx.doi.org/10.1016/j.det.2015.08.009
0733-8635/16/$ – see front matter

2. These disease must occur in 1 or more of the predilection areas: axillae, inframammary and intermammary folds, groin, perineal region, or buttocks. Lesions may appear elsewhere, as in ectopic HS, but the predilection areas must also be involved to make the diagnosis.
3. Chronicity and recurrence are important elements of the history. Temporary lesions initially recur in the predilection areas. The initial lesions progress to more chronic lesions and new lesions are added. Arbitrarily, 2 recurrences in 6 months has been used as a diagnostic criterion.[4]

All 3 criteria must be present for the definitive diagnosis and, because of the diagnostic requirement for recurrence and chronicity, an observation period may be necessary before the definitive diagnosis is made. If, for example, there is no history of recurrence and chronicity, there may be some delay in the diagnosis, which should not exceed 6 months by definition.

Several other factors may support the diagnosis but are not pathognomonic or part of the clinical definition. Familial history of HS, recurrent inflammatory uncharacteristic lesions (eg, folliculitis, open comedones) in a typical location, typical lesions in atypical location (usually pressure points and locations of enhanced mechanical friction, such as thighs or belt region of the abdomen), presence or history of a pilonidal sinus, and absence of pathogenic microbes on routine culture.

The clear clinical presentation (painful lesions recognized by patients as boils), the easily defined areas that must be affected, and the recurrent and chronic nature of the disease are sufficient for self-reported diagnosis, with a sensitivity of 90% and a specificity of 97%.[5]

OUTCOMES

Morbidity is assessed in 3 ways.

Clinical Assessment

Two types of disease severity markers are evaluated:

1. The physical signs, that is, cutaneous changes due to the disease (eg, inflamed nodules and scars)
2. An activity index (number of nodules, abscess, importance of pain, and suppuration) at a point in time or over a specified period.

These 2 aspects of morbidity are not necessarily correlated and may, in consequence, not follow a parallel evolution, suggesting that they need to be assessed separately.

Patient-reported Outcomes Measures

The use of patient-reported outcomes measures (PROMs) is generally acknowledged as a practical method to gauge the psychological consequences of the disease. Standard questionnaires on dermatologic quality of life, such as the Dermatology Life Quality Index and the Skindex, have been used to quantify the overall morbidity.[6–8] Similarly, visual analogue scales or numeric rating scales of pain and itch are highly relevant PROMs.[9,10]

Imaging and Biochemistry Studies

Classic clinical photography, using standardized photography, is useful for documentation of color, overall surface anatomy, and visible details. However, these poorly represent dermal and subcutaneous changes. These are better identified by high-frequency ultrasound as described by Wortsman.[11] MRI is also a suitable method, especially for the imaging of differential diagnosis, such as fistulae.

No pathognomonic test exists but disease activity may be reflected by changes in C-reactive protein levels and leukocyte counts.[12] Several other disease markers have been proposed but are neither routinely used nor generally available currently.[13,14]

CLINICAL ASSESSMENT

Hurley Staging

Proposed by Dr H Hurley in 1989[15] while describing surgical therapy, the stages are

- I: Abscess formation, single, or multiple, without sinus tracts and cicatrisation
- II: Recurrent abscesses with tract formation and cicatrisation, single or multiple, widely separated lesions
- III: Diffuse or near-diffuse involvement, or multiple interconnected tracts and abscesses across the entire area.

Stage I disease is thought to be the most common.[16] Most patients presenting for treatment, however, have stage II disease.

The Hurley classification has been designed to describe the severity of involvement of 1 region for surgical purpose. It cannot be used to evaluate the severity of a whole patient. In practice, however, it is frequently used as a patient's severity index to justify decisions on treatment. The scale does not reflect the current activity of the disease. It is lacking any assessment of the inflammation inherent in the disease and, instead, focuses only on consequences of the disease, that is, late changes such as scarring and tunnels. It seems mainly useful for systematic description of the earlier disease evolution.

Sartorius Score and Modified Sartorius Score

A more dynamic HS score that includes assessments of nodules, which may be transient, was created by Sartorius and colleagues[17] and later modified and partly validated.[18,19] The original Sartorius score was based on lesion counts and included scars and pustules. In the modified Sartorius score, only major characteristic elements are counted.[17–19] These include nodules and tunnels (fistulas). In both, versions the longest distance between 2 lesions in a region is measured as a surrogate of the area involved and extra points are given to Hurley classification criteria of involvement of 3 areas.[18] The lesional counting makes the score difficult to use in cases of advanced disease in which multiple lesions merge into plaques. In contrast, mild HS can be measured comfortably in a routine clinical setting after the assessor has achieved some familiarity with the score. The modified Sartorius score is commonly used in clinical trials.

Physician Global Assessment

An HS-specific physician global assessment (PGA) containing 6 categories has been used in trials.[20] The categories describe the stages of HS:

- Clear: no inflammatory or noninflammatory nodules
- Minimal: only noninflammatory nodules are present
- Mild: fewer than 5 inflammatory nodules without abscesses and draining fistulas, or 1 abscess or draining fistula without additional inflammatory nodules
- Moderate: fewer than 5 inflammatory nodules or 1 abscess, or draining fistula and 1 or more inflammatory nodules, or 2 to 5 abscesses or draining fistulas and less than 10 inflammatory nodules
- Severe: 2 to 5 abscesses or draining fistulas and 10 or more inflammatory nodules
- Very severe: more than 5 abscesses or draining fistulas.

The PGA considers only inflammatory lesions, namely inflammatory nodules, abscesses, and fistulas. It is well adapted in clinical practice to the management of patients receiving medical treatments. The PGA has not been used to classify populations in descriptive studies.

The Hidradenitis Suppurativa Severity Index

This score is not often used, and combines categorical objective and subjective parameters. The HS Severity Index Score has been used in 2 studies of the efficacy of infliximab.[21,22]

CLINICALLY MEANINGFUL DIFFERENCES

Generally, validation of the clinical scores is incomplete, although efforts are being made to provide additional data. When using the PGA, a clinically meaningful change was defined as improvement in category, for example, from very severe to moderate. In consequence, clinically meaningful differences have not been defined.

The most successful development of a validated clinical assessment system is the HS Clinical Response (HiSCR).[23,24] The HiSCR was developed as a more dynamic and validated outcome variable based on data derived from the phase 2 study of adalimumab and based on lesion counts of transient and chronic inflamed lesions. The HiSCR is defined as a greater than or equal to 50% reduction in inflammatory (transient) lesion-count (sum of abscesses and inflammatory nodules) and no increase in abscesses or draining fistulas (chronic inflamed lesions) when compared with baseline. In other words, it is a reduction of transient inflamed lesions without a concomitant increase in chronic inflamed lesions. The results were validated through PROM and PGA data. It is mostly useful as an endpoint for therapeutic trials.

PATIENT-REPORTED OUTCOMES MEASURES

Although there is a correlation between objective or physician-assessed and patient-reported severity of disease, it is not strong and probably not linear. In addition, the correlation is probably not stable over time because patients' interindividual and intraindividual coping resources vary. Regular measurements of PROM, therefore, constitute an important aspect of disease severity assessment. Several methods are available and suitable for this.

Visual Analogue Scales or Numeric Rating Scales

The use of these generic tools to quantify patients' general assessment of disease severity, as well as specific components of HS such as pain and itch is recommended.[9,10] The simultaneous use of several PROMs allows a better assessment of current disease severity and thus treatment effect.[25]

Psychometric Scales

A significant association between HS and depression has been described, indicating that a holistic approach to the severity assessment should include screening for depression.[26–30] This may, of course, be done clinically. However, a standardized approach using a tested and validated questionnaire, such as the Beck Depression Inventory or a similar tool, has many advantages when used in routine screening.[31]

Quality of Life Measures

Standard questionnaires on dermatologic quality of life, such as the Dermatology Life Quality Index and Skindex, have been used to quantify the overall morbidity.[6,7] This is further discussed in this issue in the article by Deckers and Kimball.[8]

Because of the pain caused by active lesions, HS also seems to have an impact on more general quality of life measures, for example, causing restricted mobility. General scales, such as the EQ-5D or SF-36, may also be used. These scales are usually not sufficiently sensitive when used in skin diseases but their use allows comparisons with the general health state and disutility in a broader context.[30,32–35]

IMAGING AND BIOCHEMISTRY STUDIES

Imaging

Classic clinical photography, using standardized photography is useful for documentation of color, overall surface anatomy, and visible details; however, it poorly represents dermal and subcutaneous changes. These are better identified by high-frequency ultrasound.[11,36,37]

Biochemistry Studies

Biochemistry studies in HS patients serve a twofold purpose: the assessment of HS severity and the assessment of comorbidities. For the assessment of HS severity, several markers have been proposed in studies.[13,14] In routine use, high-sensitivity C-reactive protein and a leukocyte differential count can support decision-making and monitor progress in advanced cases.[12] The abnormalities and changes are, however, usually very small.

SUMMARY

Simple diagnostic criteria are formulated for HS based on the presence of defined elements occurring in a characteristic topography and the chronic and recurrent nature of the disease. Explicit adherence to diagnostic criteria is strongly recommended. HS has been an orphan disease because this ambiguity has not been the case in other fields of medicine and has led to significant delays in diagnosis and treatment of the patients. Furthermore, it is recommended that disease severity is assessed systematically using clinical scores and PROMs for follow-up of all cases. For severe cases, other measures, such biochemistry studies and ultrasound, should be included if available. Clinical scores should describe physical signs as well as provide an estimate of disease activity.

REFERENCES

1. Saunte DM, Boer J, Stratigos A, et al. Diagnostic Delay in Hidradenitis Suppurativa is a Global Problem. Br J Dermatol 2015. [Epub ahead of print].
2. Zouboulis CC, Desai N, Emtestam L, et al. European S1 guideline for the treatment of hidradenitis suppurativa/acne inversa. J Eur Acad Dermatol Venereol 2015;29:619–44.
3. Freysz M, Jemec GB, Lipsker D. A systematic review of terms used to describe hidradenitis suppurativa. Br J Dermatol 2015. [Epub ahead of print].
4. Vinding GR, Miller IM, Zarchi K, et al. The prevalence of inverse recurrent suppuration: a population-based study of possible hidradenitis suppurativa. Br J Dermatol 2014;170:884–9.
5. Esmann S, Dufour DN, Jemec GB. Questionnaire-based diagnosis of hidradenitis suppurativa: specificity, sensitivity and positive predictive value of specific diagnostic questions. Br J Dermatol 2010; 163:102–6.
6. Basra MK, Chowdhury MM, Smith EV, et al. A review of the use of the dermatology life quality index as a criterion in clinical guidelines and health technology assessments in psoriasis and chronic hand eczema. Dermatol Clin 2012;30:237–44, viii.DLQI.
7. Finlay AY. Quality of life assessments in dermatology. Semin Cutan Med Surg 1998;17:291–6.
8. Deckers I, Kimball AB. The handicap of hidradenitis suppurativa. Derm Clin, in press.
9. McCormack HM, Horne DJ, Sheather S. Clinical applications of visual analogue scales: a critical review. Psychol Med 1988;18:1007–19.
10. Hägermark O, Wahlgren CF. Some methods for evaluating clinical itch and their application for studying pathophysiological mechanisms. J Dermatol Sci 1992;4:55–62.
11. Wortsman X. Imaging of hidradenitis suppurativa. Derm Clin, in press.
12. van Rappard DC, Leenarts MF, Meijerink-van 't Oost L, et al. Comparing treatment outcome of infliximab and adalimumab in patients with severe hidradenitis suppurativa. J Dermatolog Treat 2012;23: 284–9.
13. Wieland CW, Vogl T, Ordelman A, et al. Myeloid marker S100A8/A9 and lymphocyte marker, soluble interleukin 2 receptor: biomarkers of hidradenitis suppurativa disease activity? Br J Dermatol 2013; 168:1252–8.

14. Matusiak Ł, Bieniek A, Szepietowski JC. Soluble interleukin-2 receptor serum level is a useful marker of hidradenitis suppurativa clinical staging. Biomarkers 2009;14:432–7.
15. Hurley H. Axillary hyperhidrosis, apocrine bromhidrosis, hidradenitis suppurativa, and familial benign pemphigus: surgical approach. In: Roenigh R, Roenigh H, editors. Dermatologic surgery. New York: Marcel Dekker; 1989. p. 729–39.
16. Canoui-Poitrine F, Revuz JE, Wolkenstein P, et al. Clinical characteristics of a series of 302 French patients with hidradenitis suppurativa, with an analysis of factors associated with disease severity. J Am Acad Dermatol 2009;61:51–7.
17. Sartorius K, Lapins J, Emtestam L, et al. Suggestions for uniform outcome variables when reporting treatment effects in hidradenitis suppurativa. Br J Dermatol 2003;149:211–3.
18. Sartorius K, Emtestam L, Jemec GB, et al. Objective scoring of hidradenitis suppurativa reflecting the role of tobacco smoking and obesity. Br J Dermatol 2009;161:831–9.
19. Sartorius K, Killasli H, Heilborn J, et al. Interobserver variability of clinical scores in hidradenitis suppurativa is low. Br J Dermatol 2010;162:1261–8.
20. Kimball AB, Kerdel F, Adams D, et al. Adalimumab for the treatment of moderate to severe Hidradenitis suppurativa: a parallel randomized trial. Ann Intern Med 2012;157:846–55.
21. Grant A, Gonzalez T, Montgomery MO, et al. Infliximab therapy for patients with moderate to severe hidradenitis suppurativa: a randomized, double-blind, placebo-controlled crossover trial. J Am Acad Dermatol 2010;62:205–17.
22. Amano M, Grant A, Kerdel FA. A prospective open-label clinical trial of adalimumab for the treatment of hidradenitis suppurativa. Int J Dermatol 2010;49: 950–5.
23. Kimball AB, Jemec GB, Yang M, et al. Assessing the validity, responsiveness and meaningfulness of the Hidradenitis Suppurativa Clinical Response (HiSCR) as the clinical endpoint for hidradenitis suppurativa treatment. Br J Dermatol 2014;171:1434–42.
24. Kimball AB, Sobell JM, Zouboulis CC, et al. HiSCR (Hidradenitis Suppurativa Clinical Response): a novel clinical endpoint to evaluate therapeutic outcomes in patients with hidradenitis suppurativa from the placebo-controlled portion of a phase 2 adalimumab study. J Eur Acad Dermatol Venereol 2015. [Epub ahead of print].
25. Cappelleri JC, Bushmakin AG. Interpretation of patient-reported outcomes. Stat Methods Med Res 2014;23:460–83.
26. Miller IM, Holzman RJ, Hamzavi I. Prevalence, risk factors, and comorbidities of hidradenitis suppurativa. Derm Clin, in press.
27. Shavit E, Dreiher J, Freud T, et al. Psychiatric comorbidities in 3207 patients with hidradenitis suppurativa. J Eur Acad Dermatol Venereol 2015;29:371–6.
28. Vazquez BG, Alikhan A, Weaver AL, et al. Incidence of hidradenitis suppurativa and associated factors: a population-based study of Olmsted County, Minnesota. J Invest Dermatol 2013;133:97–103.
29. Onderdijk AJ, van der Zee HH, Esmann S, et al. Depression in patients with hidradenitis suppurativa. J Eur Acad Dermatol Venereol 2013;27:473–8.
30. Matusiak L, Bieniek A, Szepietowski JC. Psychophysical aspects of hidradenitis suppurativa. Acta Derm Venereol 2010;90:264–8.
31. Narayana S, Wong CJ. Office-based screening of common psychiatric conditions. Med Clin North Am 2014;98:959–80.
32. Both H, Essink-Bot ML, Busschbach J, et al. Critical review of generic and dermatology-specific health-related quality of life instruments. J Invest Dermatol 2007;127:2726–39.
33. Pereira FR, Basra MK, Finlay AY, et al. The role of the EQ-5D in the economic evaluation of dermatological conditions and therapies. Dermatology 2012;225: 45–53.
34. Mikkelsen PR, Vinding GR, Ring HC, et al. Disutility in patients with hidradenitis suppurativa: a cross-sectional study using EuroQoL-5D. Acta Derm Venereol 2015. [Epub ahead of print].
35. Vinding GR, Knudsen KM, Ellervik C, et al. Self-reported skin morbidities and health-related quality of life: a population-based nested case-control study. Dermatology 2014;228(3):261–8.
36. Wortsman X, Moreno C, Soto R, et al. Ultrasound in-depth characterization and staging of hidradenitis suppurativa. Dermatol Surg 2013;39:1835–42.
37. Zarchi K, Yazdanyar N, Yazdanyar S, et al. Pain and inflammation in hidradenitis suppurativa correspond to morphological changes identified by high-frequency ultrasound. J Eur Acad Dermatol Venereol 2015;29:527–32.

Prevalence, Risk Factors, and Comorbidities of Hidradenitis Suppurativa

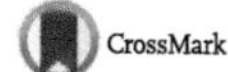

Iben Marie Miller, MD, PhD[a], Rachel J. McAndrew, MD[b], Iltefat Hamzavi, MD[c,*]

KEYWORDS

• Prevalence • Incidence • Hidradenitis suppurativa • Metabolic syndrome • Smoking • Malignancies • Spondylarthritis • Psychological comorbidities

KEY POINTS

- The true prevalence of hidradenitis suppurativa (HS) is challenging to estimate because it is often under diagnosed and misdiagnosed; the incidence seems to be increasing.
- HS is associated with a wide range of somatic comorbidities, from metabolic syndrome to rheumatologic conditions, as well as psychological comorbidities.
- The sum of somatic and psychological comorbidities places significant burden on HS patients beyond dermatologic symptoms.
- Treatment of HS needs to target dermatologic symptoms as well as possible comorbidities.

PREVALENCE AND INCIDENCE

As hidradenitis suppurativa (HS) has been an orphan disease for decades and subsequently a highly misdianogsed and underdiagnosed condition with a significant diagnose delay,[1,2] the true prevalence has been correspondingly challenging to estimate. Prevalences are reported as low as 0.00033% and as high as 4.1%.[3–8]

Prevalence estimates seem to fluctuate according to the nature of the study design, participants, and geography. A uniform pattern based on these methodologic differences present low prevalence rates in predominantly American studies performed on insurance databases, and contrasting higher prevalences in studies based on an HS diagnosis determined by physical examination or interviews/questionnaires.

In a health-insured–only US population of 15,054,519 participants, Cosmatos and colleagues[7] found an unadjusted prevalence of 0.053%. A similar low prevalence was found in the Massachusetts General Hospital Database.[9]

In contrast, a Danish study based on HS symptomatology in 100 females from the staff or patients referred to Department of Dermatology reported a prevalence of 4%.[5] A similar point prevalence of 4.1% was described in Danish study based on physical examination of 507 patients undergoing screening for sexually transmitted diseases.[4]

Questionnaires aimed at diagnosing HS using simple descriptions of symptoms, for example, boils and location of the boils, suggest a specificity and sensitivity of 82% to 97% and 90% to 97%, respectively.[6,10] A French population-based questionnaire study of 10,000 participants found a prevalence of 1%,[8] and a more recent Danish population study of 17,454 participants from the general population reported a prevalence of 2.1%.[6]

[a] Department of Dermatology, Roskilde Hospital, Koegevej 7-3, Roskilde 4000, Denmark; [b] Department of Dermatology, Henry Ford Hospital, Detroit, MI 48202, USA; [c] Department of Dermatology, Multicultural Dermatology Center, Henry Ford Hospital, Detroit, MI 48202, USA
* Corresponding author.
E-mail address: ihamzav1@hfhs.org

Dermatol Clin 34 (2016) 7–16
http://dx.doi.org/10.1016/j.det.2015.08.002
0733-8635/16/$ – see front matter

The incidence of HS based on an American database has been suggested to be 6 per 100,000 person-years, and seem to be increasing.[11] Thus, an increase from 4.3 per 100,000 (during 1970–1979) to 9.6 per 100,000 (during 2000–2008) was noted.[11]

RISK FACTORS AND COMORBIDITIES

There is a considerable overlap between what are characterized risk factors and comorbidities. One possible definition of a risk factor is something that increases a person's chances of developing a disease, whereas a comorbidity may be defined as a coexisting medical condition or disease process, and may be categorized as psychological or somatic.

Age and Sex

The mean age of onset is the early 20s; however, HS has additionally been reported children and postmenopausal women.[8,12] Considerable literature state a decline in prevalence after the age of 55, which may reflect an age-related clinical burnout of the HS activity or hormonal changes.[6,8] Equivalently, the observation that the female:male ratio is 3:1 led to the theory of androgens playing a pathogenetic part in HS. However, investigations have failed to support this hypothesis.[5,13]

Obesity

A sizable body of literature demonstrates obesity as a paramount risk factor.[8,14–18] Recently, a cross-sectional hospital- and population-based study comparing 32 hospital-based HS subjects, 326 population-based HS subjects, and 14,851 controls (non-HS subjects) found an odds ratio (OR) for obesity (body mass index [BMI] $\geq$30 kg/m^2) of 6.38 (95% CI, 2.99–13.62) and 2.56 (95% CI, 2.00–3.28) for hospital- and population-based HS subjects, respectively, when compared with controls.[18] Correspondingly, this study found an OR for abdominal obesity of 3.62 (95% CI, 1.73–7.60) and 2.24 (95% CI, 1.78–2.82) for the hospital- and population-based HS subjects, respectively.[18] Additionally, 2 studies including 336 and 80 hospital-based HS patients compared with controls found an association of HS and BMI as well as abdominal obesity.[16,17] Ambiguous results have, however, been described.[8]

An association between BMI and the HS severity measurement Sartorius score was found in 251 HS patients implying a dose–response relationship.[15] Moreover, the higher OR reported for hospital HS subjects compared with HS subjects from the general population might reflect differences in HS severity, and therefore be supportive of the dose–response relationship.[18] Nonetheless, results remain inconsistent with regard to severity, and surprisingly some studies have reported no correlation between the severity or duration of HS and obesity.[14,16,18]

Interventional studies are limited. However, 1 study demonstrated that a weight reduction of 15% in patients with BMI of greater than 30 kg/m^2 ameliorates HS supporting a dose–response relationship.[19] Moreover, obesity was reported as a risk factor for recurrence after CO_2 laser treatment of HS patients.[20]

Some factors may aid the pathophysiologic mechanisms behind the association of obesity and HS. The adipose cells are considered an independent endocrine tissue capable of secreting proinflammatory cytokines, which may add to the chronic inflammatory state of HS. Furthermore, obesity may lead to large skin folds enhancing the warm, humid milieu and skin-to-skin contact making a mechanically dependent exacerbation or maintenance of the HS lesions.

Smoking

Various studies report an association between smoking and HS. Rates of smoking in HS patients have been noted from 42% up to 70% to 92%.[18,21,22] A German study found the odds of having HS to be 9.4 times greater in current smokers versus non/ex-smokers.[23] Additionally, a French population-based study described a link between HS and current smoking, but not prior smoking.[8] The association with smoking has also been related to clinical HS disease severity.[15] It has recently been proposed that nonsmoking and nonobesity is associated with a better chance of HS remission, and it has come to light that HS surgery combined with smoking cessation give rise to fewer or no lesions.[21] Further aiding the dose–response relationship is a study investigating the role of smoking and obesity concluding that the severity of HS is worse in previous smokers when compared with never-smokers.[15]

A relationship between cigarette smoking and inflammation has been established previously. Kurzen and colleagues[24] hypothesized on possible pathophysiologic mechanisms of smoking on HS, for example, modification in the microflora of the skin and a prolonged secretion of nicotine in sweat inducing tumor necrosis factor (TNF)-α release and follicular occlusion.

Genetics

There also seems to be a genetic component to HS, which is discussed in greater detail by

Ingram[25]. Briefly, in 1985 Fitzsimmons and colleagues[26] identified a strong family predisposition with 34% of patient relatives having the disease as well. Three subsequent studies have also observed familial associations in HS patients.[11,27,28] Through genetic investigations, an autosomal-dominant defect encoding γ-secretase has been linked to rare forms of HS.[28,29] Additionally, a mutation in the proline–serine–threonine phosphatase-interacting protein 1 (PSTPIP1) gene has been identified in the pyoderma gangrenosum (PG), acne, HS, and pyogenic arthritis (PAPASH) syndrome involving HS. This syndrome is discussed elsewhere in this article.[30–32] Mutations in this gene have also been implicated in autoinflammatory syndromes. A possible association of HS to HLA-B, HLA-DR, or CARD15 polymorphisms has not been found so far.[33,34]

Other Risk Factors

Additional risk factors associated with worsening of the HS disease activity are heat, exercise, sweating, stress, fatigue, friction, tight clothing, deodorants, other cosmetics, shaving, menstruation, and brewers yeast.[35,36] However, the body of evidence concerning these risk factors is limited.

Metabolic Comorbidities

Metabolic comorbidities involves medical conditions of, relating to, or resulting from metabolism, that is, anabolic or catabolic processes. Preceding research of metabolic comorbidities in inflammatory diseases has provided evidence of an association between the metabolic syndrome and, for example, psoriasis, rheumatoid arthritis, and systemic lupus erythematosus.[37,38]

Increasing evidence furthermore proposes HS to be associated with the metabolic syndrome.[16–18] Because the metabolic syndrome is a cluster of cardiovascular risk factors including diabetes/insulin resistance, hypertension, dyslipidemia, and obesity, there is a clear overlap between this comorbidity and the risk factors obesity and smoking.

Sabat and colleagues[16] and Gold and colleagues[17] performed hospital-based studies of 80 and 366 HS patients, respectively, and found the metabolic syndrome to be a comorbidity of HS. Gold and colleagues[17] found that 50.6% of HS patients compared with 30.2% of the controls suffered from the metabolic syndrome ($P<.001$). Equivalently, Sabat and colleagues[16] reported 40% of HS patients versus 13% of controls having the metabolic syndrome yielding an OR of 4.46 (95% CI, 2.02–9.96). A large Danish study[18] including both a population- and a hospital-based sample of 358 HS subjects confirmed these results, and demonstrated 32.2% of population-based HS subjects and 53.1% of hospital-based HS subjects versus 21.5% of controls with the metabolic syndrome resulting in a higher OR for the hospital-based HS subjects (OR, 3.89 [95% CI, 1.90–7.98] vs OR, 2.08 [95% CI, 1.61–2.69]). Because hospital-based HS subjects may have a more severe degree of HS, these results may advocate a dose–response relationship and, according to Hills causal criteria, this could favor a possible causal relation. Even so, all studies so far have been observational and subsequently cannot prove causality.

Possible pathophysiologic mechanisms behind the supposed association of HS and the metabolic syndrome introduce a hypothesis concerning the long-term effects of the chronic inflammatory state of HS, the sedentary lifestyle (ie, overeating, lack of physical exercise) that may accompany HS patients as a consequence of psychological stigmatization, inflammation-induced neuropsychological factors affecting appetite and cortisone levels, and concomitant pharmacotherapy with subsequent increased cardiovascular risk.

Autoimmune Comorbidities

There is significant overlap between patients with HS and inflammatory bowel disease (IBD), especially Crohn's disease (CD).[39] A recent cross-sectional study of 1093 patients with IBD found that 255 of these patients (23%) also had HS.[40] More specifically, 26% of those with CD and 18% of ulcerative colitis patients also had HS.[40] Similar findings were reported by these authors in their 2010 evaluation of 158 IBD patients.[41]

Further complicating the matter is the fact that differentiating cutaneous CD from HS may prove difficult. Jemec and colleagues[42] described lesions in CD to be more ulcerative, the scars more retractile, and largely confined to the anorectal skin and initial rectal mucosa. However, these lesions commonly extend to create fistulas, strictures, and even incontinence when the anal sphincter is involved. HS lesions, on the other hand, do not form endoanal lesions or primary ulcerations. Comedones, nodules, skin bridging, and sinuses are present instead.[42] Physical examination should be adequate to distinguish these 2 entities in most cases, but MRI may be useful for some cases of perianal IBD versus HS.[42] It should also be noted that patients can have both HS and IBD. In both IBD studies mentioned, van der Zee and colleagues did not ask about involvement of the perianal area to avoid confusion with cutaneous perianal lesions associated with CD, so these studies may actually underrepresent the number of IBD patients with HS.

One retrospective study of 61 HS cases found 24 patients (38%) also had a diagnosis of CD.[43] On average, the diagnosis of CD predated the diagnosis of HS by 3.5 years.[43] Another study including 37 cases of HS and CD also found the diagnosis of CD usually predated HS,[44] and it was speculated that, because both CD and HS have compromised barriers (cutaneous and intestinal), an abnormal immune response from pathogen exposure or genetics may be involved.[44]

PG is a rare inflammatory condition that commonly presents as a painful nodule on the lower extremity before breaking down to an ulcer with a raised, undermined border.[45] PG has known associations with IBD, inflammatory arthritis, and myeloproliferative disorders.[45] Furthermore, several syndromes with PG and HS have been named: PASH (PG, acne conglobata, and HS), PAPASH (PG, acne, HS, and pyogenic arthritis), and PASS (PG, acne conglobata, HS, and axial spondyloarthopathy).

To date, 33 nonsyndromic cases of PG and HS have been described in the literature. Eleven of these cases were reported in a 2010 multicenter, retrospective study.[45] Interestingly, the onset of HS predated PG in all patients with a mean time of 2.5 years prior. Additionally, the mean onset of HS before PG in 20 cases in the literature before 2010 was found be 19 years.[45–53] The average age for each disease onset was 24 and 43 years, respectively.

Three PG and HS syndromes are reported in the literature. Each of these syndromes consists of the triad of PG, acne conglobata, and HS, and are be differentiated clinically by their arthritic component: PAPASH (pyogenic arthritis), PASS (seronegative spondyloarthritis), and PASH (no arthritis).[54,55] Genetically, PASS seems to be a distinct condition with no gene mutations identified. PAPASH and PASH may share a common underlying pathophysiology, because a missense mutation (c.831G→T nucleotide substitution) in the PSTPIP1 gene and increased number of microsatellite repeats in the PSTPIP1 promoter region has been found in each syndrome, respectively.[30,32] PSTPIP1 gene mutations have also been described in PAPA syndrome (triad of PG, acne conglobata, and pyogenic arthritis) and familial Mediterranean fever (an autoinflammatory disorder).[56]

PSTPIP1 regulates immune activation through its interaction with pyrin. Pyrin downregulates the immune system by decreasing interleukin (IL)-1β production that, in turn, decreases subsequent production and release of several inflammatory cytokines. When mutated, PSTPIP1 seems to exert a dominant-negative effect on pyrin, increasing IL-1β and neutrophil-mediated inflammation.[31,56] Thus, patients with PASH syndrome have significantly greater expression of cutaneous IL-1β and its receptors I and II (P = .028, .047, and .050, respectively) compared with controls.[31] Interestingly, PASH's serum inflammatory markers do not seem to be elevated, indicating that the inflammatory process in PASH is mainly localized in the skin.[31] Reports of patients with PASH treated with the IL-1 receptor antagonist (IL-1RA), anakinra, have shown mixed results.[57–59] Thus, IL-1RA may only confer partial blockage of IL-1β.[59] Further investigation on the utility of IL-1RA in PASH syndrome is warranted.

In addition to IL-1β, recent findings indicate a possible role of IL-17 in PASH. In Garzorz and colleagues'[55] report on a patient with PASH and psoriasis, 2 punch biopsies (one consistent with psoriasis, the other with PG) revealed a prominent infiltrate of IL-17–positive immune cells by immunohistochemistry. Following initiation of a TNF-α inhibitor, IL-17 and IL-22 levels were found to be 5 times greater than those of health controls. Although these results could be driven solely by the patient's psoriasis, the utility of future IL-17 blockers in patients with variants of PASH/PAPASH syndrome should not be excluded.

Follicular Occlusion Triad, Acne, and Syndromes

The basic etiopathogenesis of HS has been partly attributed to follicular occlusion from infundibular hyperkeratosis and follicular epithelium hyperplasia.[60,61] This occlusion incites perifollicular inflammation and follicular rupture, leading to the formation of the cysts, abscesses, and sinus tracts that define the clinical pathology of HS.[61] In addition to HS, follicular occlusion is an etiologic factor in acne conglobata and dissecting cellulitis of the scalp as well. Kierland[62] first described the concurrence of these 3 conditions in 1951 as the follicular occlusion triad. Shortly thereafter, Brunsting[63] highlighted commonalities between the conditions, including hyperplasia of the pilosebaceous apparatus, follicular occlusion, bacterial invasion with suppuration, and cicatricial healing. In 2013, subtypes for HS were described following Latent Class modeling (LC): LC1 being axillary–mammary, LC2 as follicular, and LC3 as gluteal.[64]

There are several cases in the literature citing the coincidence of follicular occlusion disorders in the same patient.[65–68] More recently, pilonidal sinuses have been recognized to accompany this group of follicular occlusion disorders, creating the follicular occlusion tetrad: HS, acne conglobata, dissecting cellulitis, and pilonidal cysts.[69]

Acne vulgaris has also been associated with HS. In an American and a French study 36.2% and 27.7% of HS patients seemed to suffer from acne, respectively.[11,14] In addition, there have been reports of HS associated with keratitis–ichthyosis–deafness syndrome.[70–72] One patient exhibited congenital deafness, palmoplanta keratoderma, itchthyosiform scaling, follicular hyperkeratosis, and mild keratitis in addition to dissecting cellulitis of the scalp, cystic acne, and HS.[70] In this patient, genetic analysis revealed a point mutation in a gap junction protein, connexin 26. This demonstrated a potential genetic link between these 2 syndromes, because mutations in connexin 26 have been involved in syndromes associated with both sensorineural deafness and hyperkeratotic skin disorders.[70,73] It is likely that the abnormal keratinization associated with keratitis–ichthyosis–deafness syndrome leads to the follicular plugging seen in follicular occlusion disorders.

Dowling–Degos disease is an autosomal dominantly inherited genodermatosis that presents with spotted, reticular pigmentation on the flexural surfaces.[74] Dowling–Degos disease is also related to follicular plugging and the coexistence of these conditions may be explained by the commonly shared pathogenesis of follicular occlusion as well as the distribution on the body.[75] One case series in 1993 found that 8 of 21 patients (38.1%) with Dowling–Degos disease also had HS.[76] Additionally, 6 other cases have described this association.[74,75,77–80] Last, scarce literature has proposed a link between HS and Down syndrome.[81]

Rheumatologic Comorbidities

An association between rheumatologic joint conditions, namely spondyloarthopathies and synovitis, arthritis, pustulosis, hyperostosis, osteitis (SAPHO) syndrome has been seen in conjunction with HS. Similar to the theory of pathogenesis related to antigenic exposure from compromised physical barriers, Jemec and colleagues[42] proposed that the development of these rheumatologic comorbidities may be owing to cutaneous antigen exposure that is not usually encountered systemically. These antigens may induce inflammation and antibody complexes that get deposited in the synovial fluid, inciting inflammatory, sterile arthropathy.

Spondyloarthropathies were first described by Wright[82] in 1978 as a group of seronegative (negative rheumatoid factor) arthropathies including psoriatic arthritis, ankylosing spondylitis, arthritis of IBD, and reactive arthritis. The commonalities between these spondyloarthropathies include being seronegative with sacroiliitis/spondylitis, peripheral mono/polyarthritis, genetic predisposition, and extraarticular manifestations of the skin, mucous membranes, eyes, and internal organs.[82,83] Although the first association of HS and spondyloarthropathies was reported in 1978, it took approximately 30 years before a prospective evaluation of this association was published.[51,84] This prospective evaluation was performed as a multicenter, observational study of 640 patients with HS.[84] Consistent with much of the HS demographic data, the study population had a mean age of 39.4 years, 80% female, 70% current smokers, and the mean BMI was 29.4 kg/m^2, and the distribution of Hurley stages were 16% I, 38% II, and 44% III.[84] Of the 640 HS patients, 184 (28.8%) had musculoskeletal symptoms, 43 (6.9%) had evidence of arthritis, enthesitis, or inflammatory back pain, and 24 (3.7%) were diagnosed with spondyloarthropathy after evaluation by x-ray, MRI, and a rheumatologist. Of patients with both HS and joint pain, the HS preceded joint pain in 90% of cases by a mean of 3.6 years. Of arthritic patients also assessed for HLA-B27, 9 of 16 (56.3%) were HLA-B27 negative.

In a retrospective study of 29 cases of HS and spondyloarthropathy, involvement of axial (69%) and peripheral (86%) joints was common.[67] The knee was the most frequently affected peripheral joint (59%).[67] In a prospective study of 44 patients with HS and seronegative spondyloarthropathy, there were no differences in HLA antigen frequencies compared with a control group.[85] A prior case series on these conditions reported axial joint involvement in 10 of 10 cases, peripheral joint involvement in 8 of 10 cases, and cutaneous manifestations preceding arthritic symptoms in 8 of 10 cases.[51]

The diagnosis of SAPHO syndrome includes: (1) sterile acute or chronic joint inflammation with (a) pustolosis, (b) acne, or (c) hidrandenitis suppurativa; (2) multifocal, noninfectious osteomyelitis; (3) sterile monoosteitis or polyosteitis.[50] In SAPHO, it is thought that chronic exposure to common cutaneous bacterial agents may promote desensitization, permitting low virulence infection or artherogenic stimulants resulting in arthritis and osteitis for genetically susceptible individuals.[44,84]

In a prospective HS study from Richette and associates,[84] 4 of 640 patients (0.63%) were identified as having SAPHO. The prevalence of SAPHO in the general population has never been characterized, but estimates are around 0.01% to 0.04%.[86] In 2002, Steinhoff and colleagues[50] reported a case series of 12 patients with SAPHO and 7 (58.3%) also had HS. Additional cases of these comorbid conditions have been reported in the literature.[87,88]

Malignancies

Concern for HS-associated malignancies first arose from the discovery of squamous cell carcinomas (SCC) within or neighboring HS lesions in 3.1% to 3.2% of evaluated HS patients.[89,90] A retrospective study of 2119 patients with HS found a 50% increased risk of cancer of all types compared with the standard incidence of cancer in the Swedish population being studied.[91] Specifically, nonmelanoma skin cancer, buccal cancer, and primary liver cancer were significantly increased in these patients. However, the authors did note that buccal and liver cancers might be disproportionately increased owing to uncontrolled confounders.[91] Given the significantly elevated risk of nonmelanoma skin cancer arising in HS lesions, examiners should raise their index of suspicion for malignancy and lower their biopsy threshold in HS patients to prevent or minimize SCC metastasis.

In 2011, Losanoff and colleagues[92] reviewed 64 cases of SCC arising in HS and reported 2 new cases. They found that most SCCs were diagnosed 20 to 30 years after HS and the prevalence varied by anatomic distribution: 37% gluteal, 29% perianal, 21% perineal, 10% thigh, and 3% groin and trunk. No cases have been reported in the axilla.[92,93]

Scheinfeld[93] proposes that the development of malignancy occurs owing to a synergistic effect between the chronic inflammation of HS, impaired cellular immunity, and the presence of the human papillomavirus. Chronic inflammation is associated with malignant transformation in a number of other conditions (eg, Crohns disease, Marjolin's ulcers), and thus could be a contributory factor to the development of SCCs in HS.[94,95] Prolonged inflammation, decreased tumor suppressor activity, and decreased innate immunity in HS skin are likely causative factors.[96,97] One case series of HS lesions had positive human papillomavirus test in all 8 cases evaluated; 7 of these 8 cases were positive for the high-risk subtype, human papillomavirus-16.[98] After the use of biologics in the management of HS, additional concerns regarding precipitating the development of SCC have developed.[93] However, it is unclear whether or not there is a causal relationship. A metaanalysis of 74 randomized controlled trials with anti–TNF-α biologics failed to confirm or refute that short-term anti–TNF-α agents caused an increase in the development of malignancy.[99]

Other Somatic Complications

Additional complications to HS have been suggested, for example, anemia, amyloid, and most recently renal hyperfiltration.[100–103]

PSYCHOLOGICAL COMORBIDITIES

Because the skin is a visible and a communicative organ, having a skin disease may subsequently advocate psychological comorbidities. Quality of life, which is a broad term, has been found to be impaired in HS in an even greater extent than diseases like psoriasis, acne, neoplasms, strokes, or even heart transplant candidates when investigated by general quality of life questionnaires such as EuroQol-5D and dermatology-specific questionnaires such as Dermatology Life Quality Index.[29,104,105]

There is significant evidence that HS carries a high incidence of depression.[11,106] Using a database with more than 4.1 million patients, Shavit and colleagues[107] identified 3207 HS patients diagnosed by a dermatologist and compared them against 6412 age- and gender-matched controls. In this HS cohort, 5.9% and 3.9% of patients had a diagnosis of depression and anxiety, respectively. These prevalences were significantly higher than controls ($P<.001$). Higher rates of diagnosed depression (48.1% and 42.9%) were reported in 2 cross-sectional analyses with 154 and 255 HS patients, respectively.[11,108] In 54 HS patients screened for depression using the Beck Depression Inventory-Short Form, 19.5% patients had a score suggesting depression.[104] Additionally, HS patients seem to have more severe depression than other dermatologic patients (mean Beck Depression Inventory scores, 11.0 vs 7.2; $P<.0001$).[109]

There are several plausible connections between HS and depression. HS is chronic and recurrent condition with painful, unsightly, and malodorous lesions. The resulting physical and psychological effects of this condition can disable some and lead to feelings of embarrassment with subsequent social isolation in many more.[110] Additionally, studies have recognized an association between depression and inflammation. Kurek and colleagues[111] found a significant association between HS disease severity, inflammation (as measured by C-reactive protein levels), and depression, thus highlighting the need for early management interventions, which may slow disease progression and decrease the systemic inflammation and debilitating symptoms that lead to psychological comorbidity.

An additional contributor to impaired quality of life may be the influence of HS on intimate relationships and sexual activity. The body of literature in this field is scarce. However, a German study of 24 women and 20 men suggested HS to be associated with sexual dysfunction.[112] In line with this, qualitative interviews focusing on intimate relationships reported psychological distress in HS patients dating or early in a relationship owing to embarrassment over scars and deformations created by HS, and some patients revealed that their sexual life stopped altogether owing to HS.[110] Although HS seems to burden intimate relationships, a study found that 73.5% of affected patients do in fact find a partner.[6]

The sum of psychological comorbidities may be owing to a mix of psychological stigmatization concerning the negative connotations of boils, psychological distress owing to HS-related pain, suppuration, and smell, as well as additional somatic comorbidities such as the metabolic syndrome and somatic complications of the chronic inflammation.

SUMMARY

The true prevalence of HS is challenging to estimate because it is strikingly misdiagnosed and underdiagnosed. HS is associated with a number of somatic as well as psychological comorbidities that burden the HS patients beyond their skin symptoms. When treating HS patients, it is imperative to address the screening and treatment of possible comorbidities in addition to the skin symptoms.

REFERENCES

1. Mebazaa A, El AM, Zidi W, et al. Metabolic syndrome in Tunisian psoriatic patients: prevalence and determinants. J Eur Acad Dermatol Venereol 2011;25:705–9.
2. Saunte DM, Boer J, Stratigos A, et al. Diagnostic delay in hidradenitis suppurativa is a global problem. Br J Dermatol 2015. [Epub ahead of print].
3. Lookingbill DP. Yield from a complete skin examination. Findings in 1157 new dermatology patients. J Am Acad Dermatol 1988;18:31–7.
4. Jemec GB, Heidenheim M, Nielsen NH. The prevalence of hidradenitis suppurativa and its potential precursor lesions. J Am Acad Dermatol 1996;35: 191–4.
5. Jemec GB. The symptomatology of hidradenitis suppurativa in women. Br J Dermatol 1988;119: 345–50.
6. Vinding GR, Miller IM, Zarchi K, et al. The prevalence of inverse recurrent suppuration: a population-based study of possible hidradenitis suppurativa. Br J Dermatol 2014;170:884–9.
7. Cosmatos I, Matcho A, Weinstein R, et al. Analysis of patient claims data to determine the prevalence of hidradenitis suppurativa in the United States. J Am Acad Dermatol 2013;69:819.
8. Revuz JE, Canoui-Poitrine F, Wolkenstein P, et al. Prevalence and factors associated with hidradenitis suppurativa: results from two case-control studies. J Am Acad Dermatol 2008;59:596–601.
9. Sung S, Kimball AB. Counterpoint: analysis of patient claims data to determine the prevalence of hidradenitis suppurativa in the United States. J Am Acad Dermatol 2013;69:818–9.
10. Esmann S, Dufour DN, Jemec GB. Questionnaire-based diagnosis of hidradenitis suppurativa: specificity, sensitivity and positive predictive value of specific diagnostic questions. Br J Dermatol 2010;163:102–6.
11. Vazquez BG, Alikhan A, Weaver AL, et al. Incidence of hidradenitis suppurativa and associated factors: a population-based study of Olmsted County, Minnesota. J Invest Dermatol 2013;133:97–103.
12. Palmer RA, Keefe M. Early-onset hidradenitis suppurativa. Clin Exp Dermatol 2001;26:501–3.
13. Barth JH, Layton AM, Cunliffe WJ. Endocrine factors in pre- and postmenopausal women with hidradenitis suppurativa. Br J Dermatol 1996;134: 1057–9.
14. Canoui-Poitrine F, Revuz JE, Wolkenstein P, et al. Clinical characteristics of a series of 302 French patients with hidradenitis suppurativa, with an analysis of factors associated with disease severity. J Am Acad Dermatol 2009;61:51–7.
15. Sartorius K, Emtestam L, Jemec GB, et al. Objective scoring of hidradenitis suppurativa reflecting the role of tobacco smoking and obesity. Br J Dermatol 2009;161:831–9.
16. Sabat R, Chanwangpong A, Schneider-Burrus S, et al. Increased prevalence of metabolic syndrome in patients with acne inversa. PLoS One 2012;7: e31810.
17. Gold DA, Reeder VJ, Mahan MG, et al. The prevalence of metabolic syndrome in patients with hidradenitis suppurativa. J Am Acad Dermatol 2014;70:699–703.
18. Miller IM, Ellervik C, Vinding GR, et al. Association of metabolic syndrome and hidradenitis suppurativa. JAMA Dermatol 2014;150:1273–80.
19. Kromann CB, Ibler KS, Kristiansen VB, et al. The influence of body weight on the prevalence and severity of hidradenitis suppurativa. Acta Derm Venereol 2014;94:553–7.
20. Mikkelsen PR, Dufour DN, Zarchi K, et al. Recurrence rate and patient satisfaction of CO_2 laser

evaporation of lesions in patients with hidradenitis suppurativa: a retrospective study. Dermatol Surg 2015;41:255–60.
21. Kromann CB, Deckers IE, Esmann S, et al. Risk factors, clinical course and long-term prognosis in hidradenitis suppurativa: a cross-sectional study. Br J Dermatol 2014;171:819–24.
22. Kurzen H. Chirurgische behandlung der Acne Inversa an der Universitet Heidelberg. Coloproctology 2000;22:76–80.
23. Konig A, Lehmann C, Rompel R, et al. Cigarette smoking as a triggering factor of hidradenitis suppurativa. Dermatology 1999;198:261–4.
24. Kurzen H, Kurokawa I, Jemec GB, et al. What causes hidradenitis suppurativa? Exp Dermatol 2008;17:455–6 [discussion: 457–72].
25. Ingram. The genetics of Hidradenitis Suppurativa. Dermatol Clin 2016;34(1):23–8.
26. Fitzsimmons JS, Guilbert PR, Fitzsimmons EM. Evidence of genetic factors in hidradenitis suppurativa. Br J Dermatol 1985;113:1–8.
27. Matusiak L, Bieniek A, Szepietowski JC. Hidradenitis suppurativa and associated factors: still unsolved problems. J Am Acad Dermatol 2009; 61:362–5.
28. Pink AE, Simpson MA, Desai N, et al. Mutations in the gamma-secretase genes NCSTN, PSENEN, and PSEN1 underlie rare forms of hidradenitis suppurativa (acne inversa). J Invest Dermatol 2012;132:2459–61.
29. von der Werth JM, Jemec GB. Morbidity in patients with hidradenitis suppurativa. Br J Dermatol 2001; 144:809–13.
30. Braun-Falco M, Kovnerystyy O, Lohse P, et al. Pyoderma gangrenosum, acne, and suppurative hidradenitis (PASH)–a new autoinflammatory syndrome distinct from PAPA syndrome. J Am Acad Dermatol 2012;66:409–15.
31. Marzano AV, Ceccherini I, Gattorno M, et al. Association of pyoderma gangrenosum, acne, and suppurative hidradenitis (PASH) shares genetic and cytokine profiles with other autoinflammatory diseases. Medicine 2014;93:e187.
32. Marzano AV, Trevisan V, Gattorno M, et al. Pyogenic arthritis, pyoderma gangrenosum, acne, and hidradenitis suppurativa (PAPASH): a new autoinflammatory syndrome associated with a novel mutation of the PSTPIP1 gene. JAMA Dermatol 2013;149:762–4.
33. Lapins J, Olerup O, Emtestam L. No human leukocyte antigen-A, -B or -DR association in Swedish patients with hidradenitis suppurativa. Acta Derm Venereol 2001;81:28–30.
34. Nassar D, Hugot JP, Wolkenstein P, et al. Lack of association between CARD15 gene polymorphisms and hidradenitis suppurativa: a pilot study. Dermatology 2007;215:359.
35. von der Werth JM, Williams HC. The natural history of hidradenitis suppurativa. J Eur Acad Dermatol Venereol 2000;14:389–92.
36. Cannistra C, Finocchi V, Trivisonno A, et al. New perspectives in the treatment of hidradenitis suppurativa (surgery and brewer's yeast-exclusion diet): some clarifications. Surgery 2014;156:736.
37. Miller IM, Ellervik C, Yazdanyar S, et al. Meta-analysis of psoriasis, cardiovascular disease, and associated risk factors. J Am Acad Dermatol 2013;69:1014–24.
38. Rostom S, Mengat M, Lahlou R, et al. Metabolic syndrome in rheumatoid arthritis: case control study. BMC Musculoskelet Disord 2013;14:147.
39. Yazdanyar S, Miller IM, Jemec GB. Hidradenitis suppurativa and Crohn's disease: two cases that support an association. Acta Dermatovenerol Alp Pannonica Adriat 2010;19:23–5.
40. van der Zee HH, de Winter K, van der Woude CJ, et al. The prevalence of hidradenitis suppurativa in 1093 patients with inflammatory bowel disease. Br J Dermatol 2014;171:673–5.
41. van der Zee HH, van der Woude CJ, Florencia EF, et al. Hidradenitis suppurativa and inflammatory bowel disease: are they associated? Results of a pilot study. Br J Dermatol 2010;162:195–7.
42. Jemec GBE, Revuz J, Leyden JL. Hidradenitis suppurativa. Berlin, Germany: Springer; 2006.
43. Church JM, Fazio VW, Lavery IC, et al. The differential diagnosis and comorbidity of hidradenitis suppurativa and perianal Crohn's disease. Int J Colorectal Dis 1993;8:117–9.
44. Roussomoustakaki M, Dimoulios P, Chatzicostas C, et al. Hidradenitis suppurativa associated with Crohn's disease and spondyloarthropathy: response to anti-TNF therapy. J Gastroenterol 2003;38:1000–4.
45. Hsiao JL, Antaya RJ, Berger T, et al. Hidradenitis suppurativa and concomitant pyoderma gangrenosum: a case series and literature review. Arch Dermatol 2010;146:1265–70.
46. Ah-Weng A, Langtry JA, Velangi S, et al. Pyoderma gangrenosum associated with hidradenitis suppurativa. Clin Exp Dermatol 2005;30:669–71.
47. Moschella SL. Is there a role for infliximab in the current therapy of hidradenitis suppurativa? A report of three treated cases. Int J Dermatol 2007;46:1287–91.
48. Buckley DA, Rogers S. Cyclosporin-responsive hidradenitis suppurativa. J R Soc Med 1995;88: 289P–90P.
49. Raynor A, Askari AD. Behçet's disease and treatment with colchicine. J Am Acad Dermatol 1980;2:396–400.
50. Steinhoff JP, Cilursu A, Falasca GF, et al. A study of musculoskeletal manifestations in 12 patients with SAPHO syndrome. J Clin Rheumatol 2002;8: 13–22.

51. Rosner IA, Richter DE, Huettner TL, et al. Spondyloarthropathy associated with hidradenitis suppurative and acne conglobata. Ann Intern Med 1982;97:520–5.
52. von den Driesch P. Pyoderma gangrenosum: a report of 44 cases with follow-up. Br J Dermatol 1997;137:1000–5.
53. Powell FC, Schroeter AL, Su WP, et al. Pyoderma gangrenosum: a review of 86 patients. Q J Med 1985;55:173–86.
54. Bruzzese V. Pyoderma gangrenosum, acne conglobata, suppurative hidradenitis, and axial spondyloarthritis: efficacy of anti-tumor necrosis factor alpha therapy. J Clin Rheumatol 2012;18:413–5.
55. Garzorz N, Papanagiotou V, Atenhan A, et al. Pyoderma gangrenosum, acne, psoriasis, arthritis and suppurative hidradenitis (PAPASH)-syndrome: a new entity within the spectrum of autoinflammatory syndromes? J Eur Acad Dermatol Venereol 2014. [Epub ahead of print].
56. Shoham NG, Centola M, Mansfield E, et al. Pyrin binds the PSTPIP1/CD2BP1 protein, defining familial Mediterranean fever and PAPA syndrome as disorders in the same pathway. Proc Natl Acad Sci U S A 2003;100:13501–6.
57. Marzano AV, Ishak RS, Colombo A, et al. Pyoderma gangrenosum, acne and suppurative hidradenitis syndrome following bowel bypass surgery. Dermatology 2012;225:215–9.
58. Menis D, Maroñas-Jiménez L, Delgado-Marquez AM. Two cases of severe hidradenitis suppurativa with failure of anakinra therapy. Br J Dermatol 2015;172(3):810–1.
59. Staub J, Pfannschmidt N, Strohal R, et al. Successful treatment of PASH syndrome with infliximab, cyclosporine and dapsone. J Eur Acad Dermatol Venereol 2014. [Epub ahead of print].
60. Yu CC, Cook MG. Hidradenitis suppurativa: a disease of follicular epithelium, rather than apocrine glands. Br J Dermatol 1990;122:763–9.
61. von Laffert M, Stadie V, Wohlrab J, et al. Hidradenitis suppurativa/acne inversa: bilocated epithelial hyperplasia with very different sequelae. Br J Dermatol 2011;164:367–71.
62. Kierland RR. Unusual pyodermas (hidrosadenitis suppurativa, acne conglobata, dissecting cellulitis of the scalp). Minn Med 1951;34:319–25 [passim].
63. Brunsting HA. Hidradenitis and other variants of acne. AMA Arch Derm Syphilol 1952;65:303–15.
64. Canoui-Poitrine F, Le TA, Revuz JE, et al. Identification of three hidradenitis suppurativa phenotypes: latent class analysis of a cross-sectional study. J Invest Dermatol 2013;133:1506–11.
65. Chicarilli ZN. Follicular occlusion triad: hidradenitis suppurativa, acne conglobata, and dissecting cellulitis of the scalp. Ann Plast Surg 1987;18: 230–7.
66. Deschamps ME, Payet S, Tournadre A, et al. Efficacy of infliximab in the treatment of follicular occlusion triad. Ann Dermatol Venereol 2010;137: 546–50 [in French].
67. Bhalla R, Sequeira W. Arthritis associated with hidradenitis suppurativa. Ann Rheum Dis 1994; 53:64–6.
68. Thein M, Hogarth MB, Acland K. Seronegative arthritis associated with the follicular occlusion triad. Clin Exp Dermatol 2004;29:550–2.
69. Vasanth V, Chandrashekar BS. Follicular occlusion tetrad. Indian Dermatol Online J 2014;5:491–3.
70. Montgomery JR, White TW, Martin BL, et al. A novel connexin 26 gene mutation associated with features of the keratitis-ichthyosis-deafness syndrome and the follicular occlusion triad. J Am Acad Dermatol 2004;51:377–82.
71. Maintz L, Betz RC, Allam JP, et al. Keratitis-ichthyosis-deafness syndrome in association with follicular occlusion triad. Eur J Dermatol 2005;15:347–52.
72. Wenghoefer M, Allam JP, Novak N, et al. Surgical therapy in a patient with Keratosis-Ichthyosis-Deafness (KID) syndrome associated with follicular occlusion triad. Eur J Dermatol 2007;17:449–50.
73. Kelsell DP, Di WL, Houseman MJ. Connexin mutations in skin disease and hearing loss. Am J Hum Genet 2001;68:559–68.
74. Li M, Hunt MJ, Commens CA. Hidradenitis suppurativa, Dowling Degos disease and perianal squamous cell carcinoma. Australas J Dermatol 1997;38:209–11.
75. Loo WJ, Rytina E, Todd PM. Hidradenitis suppurativa, Dowling-Degos and multiple epidermal cysts: a new follicular occlusion triad. Clin Exp Dermatol 2004;29:622–4.
76. Balus L, Fazio M, Amantea A, et al. Dowling-Degos disease and Verneuil disease. Ann Dermatol Venereol 1993;120:705–8 [in French].
77. Fenske NA, Groover CE, Lober CW, et al. Dowling-Degos disease, hidradenitis suppurativa, and multiple keratoacanthomas. A disorder that may be caused by a single underlying defect in pilosebaceous epithelial proliferation. J Am Acad Dermatol 1991;24:888–92.
78. Weber LA, Kantor GR, Bergfeld WF. Reticulate pigmented anomaly of the flexures (Dowling-Degos disease): a case report associated with hidradenitis suppurativa and squamous cell carcinoma. Cutis 1990;45:446–50.
79. Bedlow AJ, Mortimer PS. Dowling-Degos disease associated with hidradenitis suppurativa. Clin Exp Dermatol 1996;21:305–6.
80. Choudhary SV, Jain D, Agrawal P, et al. Dowling-Degos disease and hidradenitis suppurativa: co occurrence or association? Indian Dermatol Online J 2013;4:191–4.
81. Blok J, Jonkman M, Horvath B. The possible association of hidradenitis suppurativa and Down

syndrome: is increased amyloid precursor protein expression resulting in impaired Notch signalling the missing link? Br J Dermatol 2014;170:1375–7.
82. Wright V. Seronegative polyarthritis: a unified concept. Arthritis Rheum 1978;21:619–33.
83. Muller W. Seronegative rheumatic spondyloarthropathies (spondarthritis). Schweiz Med Wochenschr 1982;112:1262–72 [in German].
84. Richette P, Molto A, Viguier M, et al. Hidradenitis suppurativa associated with spondyloarthritis – results from a multicenter national prospective study. J Rheumatol 2014;41:490–4.
85. Rosner IA, Burg CG, Wisnieski JJ, et al. The clinical spectrum of the arthropathy associated with hidradenitis suppurativa and acne conglobata. J Rheumatol 1993;20:684–7.
86. Nguyen MT, Borchers A, Selmi C, et al. The SAPHO syndrome. Semin Arthritis Rheum 2012;42:254–65.
87. Ozyemisci-Taskiran O, Bolukbasi N, Gogus F. A hidradenitis suppurativa related SAPHO case associated with features resembling spondylarthropathy and proteinuria. Clin Rheumatol 2007;26:789–91.
88. Legrand E, Audran M, Rousselet-Chapeau MC, et al. Iliac osteosarcoma in a patient with SAPHO syndrome. Rev Rhum Engl Ed 1995;62:139–41.
89. Jackman RJ. Hidradenitis suppurativa: diagnosis and surgical management of perianal manifestations. Proc R Soc Med 1959;52(Suppl):110–2.
90. Anderson MJ Jr, Dockerty MB. Perianal hidradenitis suppurativa; a clinical and pathologic study. Dis Colon Rectum 1958;1:23–31.
91. Lapins J, Ye W, Nyren O, et al. Incidence of cancer among patients with hidradenitis suppurativa. Arch Dermatol 2001;137:730–4.
92. Losanoff JE, Sochaki P, Khoury N, et al. Squamous cell carcinoma complicating chronic suppurative hydradenitis. Am Surg 2011;77:1449–53.
93. Scheinfeld N. A case of a patient with stage III familial hidradenitis suppurativa treated with 3 courses of infliximab and died of metastatic squamous cell carcinoma. Dermatol Online J 2014;20(3).
94. Thomas M, Bienkowski R, Vandermeer TJ, et al. Malignant transformation in perianal fistulas of Crohn's disease: a systematic review of literature. J Gastrointest Surg 2010;14:66–73.
95. Sadegh Fazeli M, Lebaschi AH, Hajirostam M, et al. Marjolin's ulcer: clinical and pathologic features of 83 cases and review of literature. Med J Islam Repub Iran 2013;27:215–24.
96. Pink AE, Simpson MA, Desai N, et al. gamma-Secretase mutations in hidradenitis suppurativa: new insights into disease pathogenesis. J Invest Dermatol 2013;133:601–7.
97. Dreno B, Khammari A, Brocard A, et al. Hidradenitis suppurativa: the role of deficient cutaneous innate immunity. Arch Dermatol 2012;148:182–6.
98. Lavogiez C, Delaporte E, Darras-Vercambre S, et al. Clinicopathological study of 13 cases of squamous cell carcinoma complicating hidradenitis suppurativa. Dermatology 2010;220:147–53.
99. Askling J, Fahrbach K, Nordstrom B, et al. Cancer risk with tumor necrosis factor alpha (TNF) inhibitors: meta-analysis of randomized controlled trials of adalimumab, etanercept, and infliximab using patient level data. Pharmacoepidemiol Drug Saf 2011;20:119–30.
100. Miller I, Carlson N, Ellervik C. A population and hospital based study of renal function in hidradentis suppurativa. Acta Derm Venereol 2014. [Epub ahead of print].
101. Tennant F Jr, Bergeron JR, Stone OJ, et al. Anemia associated with hidradenitis suppurativa. Arch Dermatol 1968;98:138–40.
102. Girouard SD, Falk RH, Rennke HG, et al. Hidradenitis suppurativa resulting in systemic amyloid A amyloidosis: a case report and review of the literature. Dermatol Online J 2012;18:2.
103. Deckers IE, van der Zee HH, Prens EP. Severe fatigue based on anaemia in patients with hidradenitis suppurativa: report of two cases and a review of the literature. J Eur Acad Dermatol Venereol 2014. [Epub ahead of print].
104. Matusiak L, Bieniek A, Szepietowski JC. Psychophysical aspects of hidradenitis suppurativa. Acta Derm Venereol 2010;90:264–8.
105. Vinding GR, Knudsen KM, Ellervik C, et al. Self-reported skin morbidities and health-related quality of life: a population-based nested case-control study. Dermatology 2014;228:261–8.
106. Onderdijk AJ, van der Zee HH, Esmann S, et al. Depression in patients with hidradenitis suppurativa. J Eur Acad Dermatol Venereol 2013;27:473–8.
107. Shavit E, Dreiher J, Freud T, et al. Psychiatric comorbidities in 3207 patients with hidradenitis suppurativa. J Eur Acad Dermatol Venereol 2015;29:371–6.
108. Crowley JJ, Mekkes JR, Zouboulis CC, et al. Association of hidradenitis suppurativa disease severity with increased risk for systemic comorbidities. Br J Dermatol 2014;171:1561–5.
109. Matusiak L, Bieniek A, Szepietowski JC. Hidradenitis suppurativa markedly decreases quality of life and professional activity. J Am Acad Dermatol 2010;62:706–8, 8.e1.
110. Esmann S, Jemec GB. Psychosocial impact of hidradenitis suppurativa: a qualitative study. Acta Derm Venereol 2011;91:328–32.
111. Kurek A, Johanne Peters EM, Sabat R, et al. Depression is a frequent co-morbidity in patients with acne inversa. J Dtsch Dermatol Ges 2013;11:743–9, 743–50.
112. Kurek A, Peters EM, Chanwangpong A, et al. Profound disturbances of sexual health in patients with acne inversa. J Am Acad Dermatol 2012;67:422–8, 8.e1.

The Handicap of Hidradenitis Suppurativa

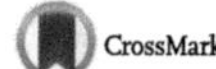

Inge Elizabeth Deckers, MD[a,*], Alexa Boer Kimball, MD, MPH[b]

KEYWORDS

• Acne inversa • Quality of life • Social impact • Depression • Psychological impact • Dermatology life quality index • Work • Morbidity

KEY POINTS

- Multiple studies have shown a diminished quality of life (QoL) in patients with hidradenitis suppurativa (HS).
- The prevalence of depression in HS ranges from 6% to 39%.
- The painful inflammation and disfiguring scars can have great impact on the sexual life of patients with HS.

INTRODUCTION

HS is a debilitating disease, because of its chronic course characterized by relapsing painful inflammatory nodules in intimate places such as the groin, pubic area, submammary area, and axillae. The inflammation not only is painful but also can cause malodorous discharge leading to soiling of cloths, and the lesions are also unsightly and deforming.[1,2] A diagnosis of HS comes with many uncertainties; the course of the disease is unknown, as is whether the disease will flare up or if patients ever will be free of inflammation. There remains a great unmet need for better therapy, and as of today, a cure is distant. Combining these factors, it is hardly surprising that HS has a negative impact on the QoL of patients.[1,3] Even though the impact of HS has gained more attention recently, only a dozen articles have been published on this subject, most of which have occurred in the past 5 years. Ingram and colleagues[4] investigated which topics should get priority in research in the next few years. The topic "the impact of HS and its treatment on people with HS (physical, psychological, financial, social, quality of life)" ranked third, confirming that the handicap of HS should gain substantially more attention in current research.

With these limitations in mind, in this article the authors give an overview of the known impact of HS on QoL, the prevalence of depression, and the influence on the sexual life and work of patients with HS.

QUALITY OF LIFE

HS can have a profound influence on QoL. Owing to pain, patients are unable to perform their everyday tasks, go to work, or enjoy sports. In addition, patients feel often embarrassed because of the malodorous inflammation and often hide the disease even from close relatives.[3]

Dermatology-Specific Quality of Life Questionnaires

QoL is generally assessed using questionnaires. There are 2 commonly used specific dermatologic

Disclosure: I.E. Deckers has no conflicts of interest to declare regarding the contents of this article; A.B. Kimball is a consultant and investigator for Abbvie, Amgen, Janssen, and Novartis and had Fellowship funding from Novartis and Janssen.

[a] Department of Dermatology, Erasmus MC, University Medical Center Rotterdam, Burgemeester s' Jacobplein 51, 3015 CA, Rotterdam, The Netherlands; [b] Department of Dermatology, Harvard Medical School, 50 Staniford Street, #240, Boston, MA 021441, USA

* Corresponding author.

E-mail address: i.deckers@erasmusmc.nl

Dermatol Clin 34 (2016) 17–22

http://dx.doi.org/10.1016/j.det.2015.07.003

0733-8635/16/$ – see front matter

QoL questionnaires, namely, the Dermatology Life Quality Index (DLQI) and the Skindex-29.

The DLQI was published in 1994 by Finlay and Khan[5] and consists of 10 questions concerning symptoms and feelings, daily activities, leisure, work and school, personal relationships, and treatment. Patients can answer with "not at all," "a little," "a lot," or "very much," resulting in a score from 0 to 3 for every question. A total score of 0 to 1 indicates no effect on QoL, 2 to 5 a small effect, 6 to 10 a moderate effect, 11 to 20 a very large effect, and 21 to 30 an extremely large effect.[5,6]

The Skindex-29 questionnaire consists of 29 questions about 3 domains, namely, emotions, symptoms, and functioning. An additional item addresses the side effects of medication and treatment.[7] Each item results in a score between 0 and 100. The domain scores are the average scores of the items within that domain. Cutoff scores for severe impaired health-related quality of life (HRQoL) for the specific domains are greater than or equal to 52 points on symptoms, greater than or equal to 39 on emotions, and greater than or equal to 37 on functioning. The total score can also be used, although less frequently. A total score more than 44 indicates a severe impaired HRQoL.[7]

Quality of Life in Patients with Hidradenitis Suppurativa

All studies performed on QoL in patients with HS to date report a diminished QoL. Most studies that used the DLQI report an average score between 8 and 13, indicating that HS has a moderate to very large effect on the QoL (**Fig. 1**).[3,8–11] Studies that used the Skindex-29 questionnaire showed scores between 52.6 and 59.2 for the emotional domain, 52.2 and 55.6 for symptoms, and 45.9 and 48.8 for the functional domain.[12,13] The only population-based study reported a much lower impact on QoL with a DLQI of 3.7 and a Skindex-29 total of 19.7.[14] However, they used self-reported diagnoses, based on diagnostic questions about HS, psoriasis, pimples, hand rash, atopic eczema, and chronic leg ulcers. Even though this study showed that all dermatologic patients had higher DLQI scores than the controls, with patients with HS having the highest mean score of 3.7, these scores were still substantially lower than in the hospital-based studies.[14]

Causes of Low Quality of Life in Hidradenitis Suppurativa

When examining predictors of low QoL, young age of onset and more lesions per month are associated with higher DLQI and Skindex scores, and the severity of HS is strongly associated with a lower QoL.[3,12,13] On the DLQI, Hurley stage I patients scored between 2.8 and 5.7 and Hurley stage II patients scored between 8.3 and 13.10, whereas in Hurley stage III patients, the scores ranged from 17.6 to 20.4, indicating a very large effect on the patient's QoL.[9,11] In addition, the

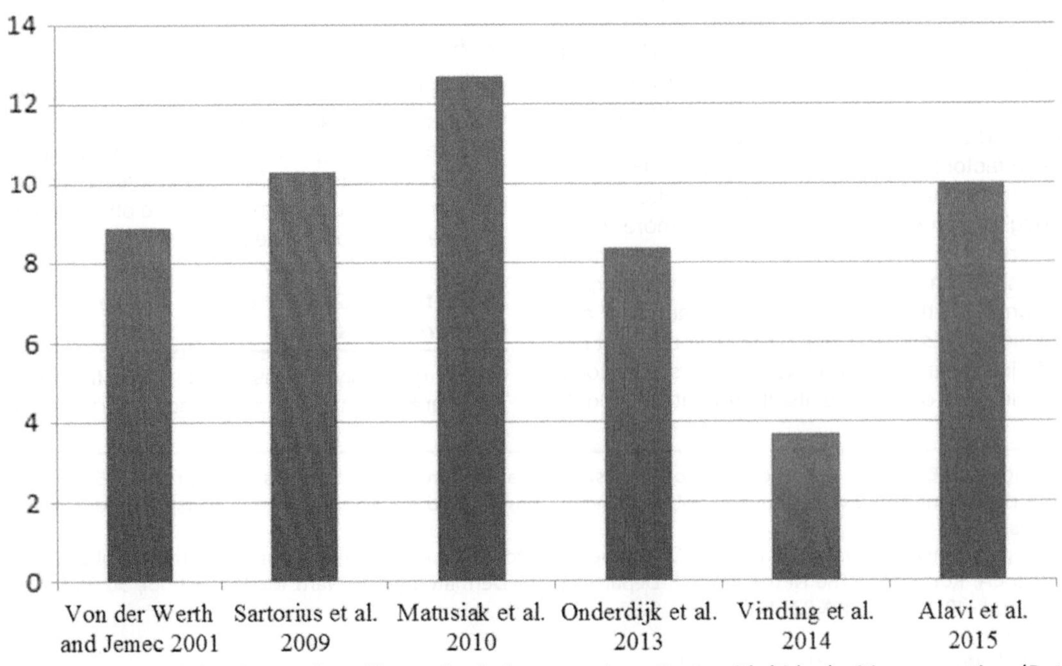

Fig. 1. Overview of the dermatology life quality index scores in patients with hidradenitis suppurativa. (*Data from* Refs.[3,8–11,14])

Sartorius score, which is used more nowadays, also showed to have a significant correlation with the DLQI scores.[8]

The DLQI questions that scored the highest were: "how itchy, sore, painful, or stinging has your skin been" and "how much has your skin influenced the clothes you wear,"[3,8,10] indicating that the pain, discomfort, and embarrassment are important factors diminishing QoL. Analyzing the Skindex-29 scores, in the symptom domain, the highest scores were obtained from items about sensitive, irritated, and painful skin. On the emotional domain, patients felt annoyed and angry about having HS and were worried that the HS would get worse. On the functional domain, fatigue scored the highest.[13] This result was consistent with that of the work by Matusiak and colleagues[9] confirming that fatigue is a prevalent problem in patients with HS. They found that almost 40% of the patients with HS had clinically significant fatigue, with a strong correlation between the Hurley stage and the level of fatigue.

Quality of Life in Hidradenitis Suppurativa Versus Other Dermatologic Diseases

In direct studies comparing DLQI scores of patients with HS with other dermatologic patients or controls, patients with HS tended to have the highest scores reported across the groups.[10,12,14] Onderdijk and colleagues[10] compared the DLQI scores of patients with HS with patients with acne, eczema, psoriasis, skin tumors, and other skin diseases and found that patients with HS had significantly higher scores than these other dermatologic patients. However, when analyzing larger-scale studies using DLQI scores in patients with skin diseases, Basra and colleagues[6] compared the DLQI scores of 45,710 patients from 220 different studies (**Fig. 2**). HS registered with a mean score of 13.3, as one of the highest. Only burns (scars) (17.8), erythropoietic protoporphyria (14.0), and hirsutism (13.4) scored higher suggesting that HS belongs in the top 5 skin diseases with the most negatively affected QoL scores.[6]

PSYCHIATRIC COMORBIDITIES

Owing to the low QoL, it is not surprising that patients with HS also more frequently suffer from psychiatric disorders. Patients report that they feel unworthy and not lovable because of the scars and ongoing inflammation.[15]

In a large database chart review using the International Classification of Diseases, Ninth Revision

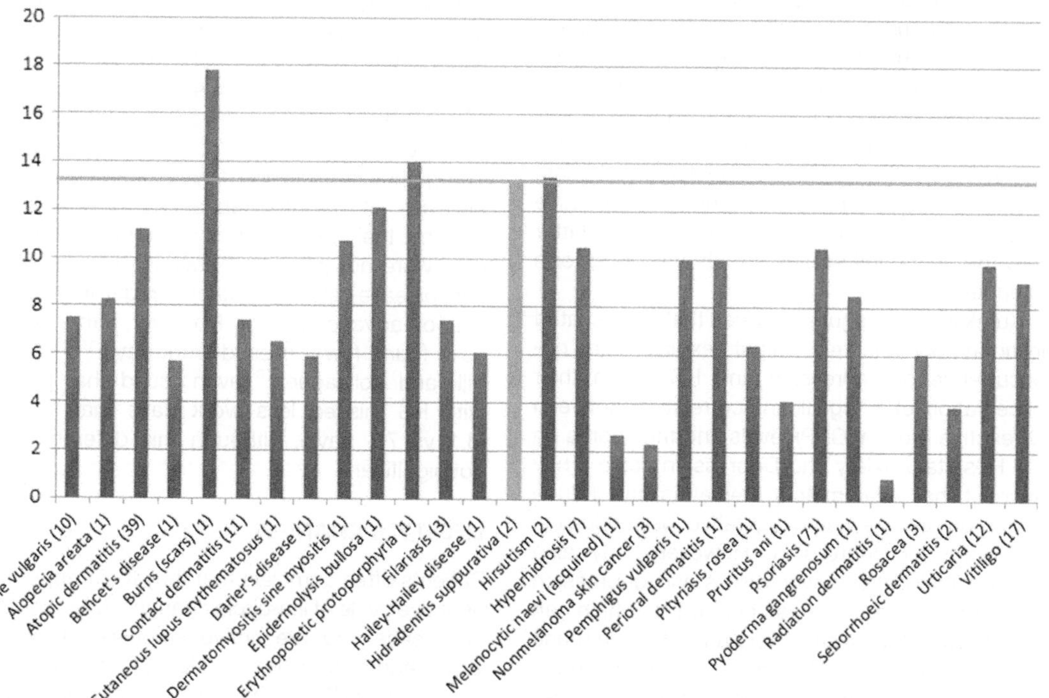

Fig. 2. An overview of the dermatology life quality index (DLQI) scores in patients with multiple different dermatologic diseases. The number of studies on which the DLQI score is based is indicated in parentheses. (*Data from* Basra MK, Fenech R, Gatt RM, et al. The dermatology life quality index 1994–2007: a comprehensive review of validation data and clinical results. Br J Dermatol 2008;159(5):997–1035.)

(ICD-9) codes, almost 60% of the patients with HS also had a diagnosis for some psychiatric disorder. After correcting for other comorbidities such as obesity, thyroid disorders, arthropathies, and diabetes, HS remained highly associated with psychiatric disorders.[16]

Depression

HS is often associated with depression but reported prevalence varies substantially across published studies. Shavit and colleagues[17] investigated the prevalence of depression in a large database including 3207 patients with HS. They found that almost 6% of the patients with HS suffered from depression. However, in questionnaire-based studies, a prevalence of depression up to 39% has been reported.[9,10,18] These findings highlight some of the differences and limitations of both administrative databases and self-reported research. Databases may underestimate prevalence because of undercoding, whereas questionnaires assessing symptoms may uncover undiagnosed conditions.

Three studies have used questionnaires to determine the prevalence of depression in HS.[9,10,18] They found a prevalence of depression between 9% and 39% in patients with HS. Unfortunately, all 3 used a different questionnaire, making direct comparison impossible.[9,10,18] In 2 studies, disease severity correlated with the depression scores.[9,18] Onderdijk and colleagues[10] could not confirm the association between depression and Hurley score, but they did find a correlation between the number of lesions and flares in the last month, which may be a better indicator of active disease than the Hurley score, because the latter may be more influenced by chronic long-term changes.

Kurek and colleagues[18] argued that the elevated inflammatory markers might explain the co-occurrence of depression and HS, given their observation of a significant correlation between C-reactive protein (CRP) levels and the scores on the Hospital Anxiety and Depression scale. They suggest that inflammatory mediators can induce and promote the neurovegetative psychological symptoms of depression. However, they also discuss that patients with stress and depression might produce more stress hormones, which can also activate the inflammatory arm of the immune system, causing a low-grade inflammation.[18] However, they ultimately found a correlation between CRP levels and the Sartorius score, strengthening the hypothesis that the primary factor driving inflammation might be the disease severity, which in turn might increase the risk of depression beyond the obvious psychosocial burden of the disease itself.

Sexual Distress

Patients often report that HS has a great influence on their sexual life. They feel embarrassed because of the inflammation and disfiguring scars often located in intimate regions. They also suffer from pain that restrains them from sexual intercourse. Patients also report that their partners lose interest in sexual activity when they have active lesions.[15]

Only one study has investigated the influence of HS on sexual health. The investigators found a significant impairment of sexual health in patients with HS compared with age-, sex-, and body mass index–matched controls.[19] Women with the same level of disease reported higher sexual distress than men, but surprisingly, there was no correlation between sexual functioning and disease severity. However, 2 patients without genital lesions had similar levels of sexual function as the healthy controls, suggesting that the location of inflammation was important in determining sexual distress.[19]

WORK

Patients often report that because of the painful lesions they are unable to go to work and sometimes even lose their jobs because of the numerous sick days. Matusiak and colleagues[20] found that patients were on average 33.6 days absent from work. Of the 30 patients, 3 reported losing their jobs in the 2-year follow-up period because of frequent absences or inability to perform their work properly. Another 7 reported they were not promoted because of their HS or had disease-related obstacles regarding promotion or advancement.[20] However, other studies have found fewer missed work days.[10,21] Onderdijk and colleagues[10] even found that patients with HS missed less work days than controls (3.1 vs 7.1 days), although this difference was not significant.

LIFESTYLE CHANGES

Patients often complain that they feel trapped in a negative cycle of life-circle changes. Most patients are obese and are active smokers.[8] However, when addressing these risk factors, they often respond that HS causes significant stress because of the painful inflammation, making it difficult to quit smoking. When they manage to quit smoking, they often start eating more, resulting in weight gain, which obviously results in more stress and feeling the need to restart smoking. Involving in sports to lose weight is often difficult because of the painful lesions. The net effect of these trade-offs can unfortunately substantially limit the ability to effect useful lifestyle changes.

HEALTH CARE COSTS

Although there is some information about the impact of HS on employment, there is little documented about the personal financial burden of patients with HS. Patients with psoriasis, in comparison, are known to spend substantially on over-the-counter supplies,[22] and this is also likely to be the case for patients with HS who use over-the-counter treatments and bandages. Only one study reported on the health care costs for patients with HS. They showed that patients with HS had significantly higher drug and pharmacy costs than patients without HS but lower costs than patients with psoriasis, probably because the latter frequently use expensive biologicals.[23] They also reported an increased use of emergency room visits and hospitalizations by patients with HS, which in some countries can also be accompanied by out-of-pocket expenditures.[23] More research in this area would be welcomed as better management and new therapies may help to control these costs.

SUMMARY

HS is a profoundly debilitating disease with a high negative impact on QoL, with multiple studies confirming that the impact is often greater than that seen with other dermatologic diseases. Patients with HS also often suffer from depression, have an impaired sexual health, and may have difficulty performing their work duties. Consistent and coordinated care with access to appropriate specialists may be an important opportunity to improve clinical outcomes, costs of care, and QoL. Providers should be aware of these implications and may be able to increase the effectiveness of their interventions with attention to these other aspects of the disease.

REFERENCES

1. Revuz JE. Hidradenitis suppurativa. J Eur Acad Dermatol Venereol 2009;23(9):985–98.
2. Alikhan A, Lynch PJ, Eisen DB. Hidradenitis suppurativa: a comprehensive review. J Am Acad Dermatol 2009;60(4):539–61.
3. Von der Werth JM, Jemec GBE. Morbidity in patients with hidradenitis suppurativa. Br J Dermatol 2001;144(4):809–13.
4. Ingram JR, Abbott R, Ghazavi M, et al. The hidradenitis suppurativa priority setting partnership. Br J Dermatol 2014;171(6):1422–7.
5. Finlay AY, Khan GK. Dermatology life quality index (DLQI)—a simple practical measure for routine clinical use. Clin Exp Dermatol 1994;19(3):210–6.
6. Basra MKA, Fenech R, Gatt RM, et al. The dermatology life quality index 1994–2007: a comprehensive review of validation data and clinical results. Br J Dermatol 2008;159(5):997–1035.
7. Prinsen CAC, Lindeboom R, Sprangers MAG, et al. Health-related quality of life assessment in dermatology: interpretation of Skindex-29 scores using patient-based anchors. J Invest Dermatol 2010;130(5):1318–22.
8. Sartorius K, Emtestam L, Jemec GBE, et al. Objective scoring of hidradenitis suppurativa reflecting the role of tobacco smoking and obesity. Br J Dermatol 2009;161(4):831–9.
9. Matusiak L, Bieniek A, Szepietowski JC. Psychophysical aspects of hidradenitis suppurativa. Acta Derm Venereol 2010;90(3):264–8.
10. Onderdijk AJ, van der Zee HH, Esmann S, et al. Depression in patients with hidradenitis suppurativa. J Eur Acad Dermatol Venereol 2013;27(4):473–8.
11. Alavi A, Anooshirvani N, Kim WB, et al. Quality-of-life impairment in patients with hidradenitis suppurativa: a Canadian study. Am J Clin Dermatol 2015;16(1):61–5.
12. Wolkenstein P, Loundou A, Barrau K, et al, Quality of Life Group of the French Society of Dermatology. Quality of life impairment in hidradenitis suppurativa: a study of 61 cases. J Am Acad Dermatol 2007;56(4):621–3.
13. Benjamins M, van der Wal VB, de Korte J. Kwaliteit van leven bij Nederlandse patiënten met hidradenitis suppurativa (acne inversa) [English abstract]. Ned Tijdschr Dermatol Venereol 2009;19:446–50.
14. Vinding GR, Knudsen KM, Ellervik C, et al. Self-reported skin morbidities and health-related quality of life: a population-based nested case-control study. Dermatology 2014;228(3):261–8.
15. Esmann S, Jemec GB. Psychosocial impact of hidradenitis suppurativa: a qualitative study. Acta Derm Venereol 2011;91(3):328–32.
16. Shlyankevich J, Chen AJ, Kim GE, et al. Hidradenitis suppurativa is a systemic disease with substantial comorbidity burden: A chart-verified case-control analysis. J Am Acad Dermatol 2014;71(6):1144–50.
17. Shavit E, Dreiher J, Freud T, et al. Psychiatric comorbidities in 3207 patients with hidradenitis suppurativa. J Eur Acad Dermatol Venereol 2015;29(2):371–6.

18. Kurek A, Peters J, Milena E, et al. Depression is a frequent co-morbidity in patients with acne inversa. J Dtsch Dermatol Ges 2013;11(8):743–9.
19. Kurek A, Peters EMJ, Chanwangpong A, et al. Profound disturbances of sexual health in patients with acne inversa. J Am Acad Dermatol 2012; 67(3):422–8.
20. Matusiak Ł, Bieniek A, Szepietowski JC. Hidradenitis suppurativa markedly decreases quality of life and professional activity. J Am Acad Dermatol 2010; 62(4):706–8.
21. Jemec GBE, Heidenheim M, Nielsen NH. Hidradenitis suppurativa - characteristics and consequences. Clin Exp Dermatol 1996;21(6):419–23.
22. Javitz HS, Ward MM, Farber E, et al. The direct cost of care for psoriasis and psoriatic arthritis in the United States. J Am Acad Dermatol 2002;46(6): 850–60.
23. Kirby JS, Miller JJ, Adams DR, et al. Health care utilization patterns and costs for patients with hidradenitis suppurativa. JAMA Dermatol 2014;150(9): 937–44.

The Genetics of Hidradenitis Suppurativa

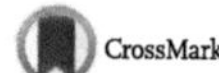

John R. Ingram, MA, MSc, DM, MRCP(Derm), FAcadMEd

KEYWORDS

- Hidradenitis suppurativa • Genetics • Gamma secretase • Notch signaling

KEY POINTS

- A family history of hidradenitis suppurativa (HS) is reported by about one-third of patients, and the pattern of inheritance suggests an autosomal dominant trait.
- Heterozygous γ-secretase gene mutations have been found in patients with HS from China, Europe, and other locations.
- γ-Secretase is a transmembrane protease involved in the Notch signaling pathway.
- Mutations of γ-secretase have been found in only a minority of patients with HS.

INTRODUCTION

In discussing the etiology of HS, potential causes can be subdivided into genetic, microbiological, endocrine, and environmental factors such as obesity and smoking. The question, "To what extent is HS caused by genetic factors?" was recently placed in the top 10 most important uncertainties from a short list of 55 HS uncertainties in a Priority Setting Partnership conducted for HS, in which patients with HS, carers, and clinicians agreed mutually important HS research questions.[1] Patients were keen to know the chances of passing on the condition to their children, and clinicians saw the opportunity to develop targeted therapies for HS by identifying the protein products of any relevant gene mutations.

CONTRIBUTION OF GENETICS TO HIDRADENITIS SUPPURATIVA ETIOLOGY

Any determination of the relative contribution of genetic and environmental factors in disease causation usually incorporates twin studies, to compare disease risk in monozygotic and dizygotic pairs. Unfortunately, twin data are currently lacking in HS. One pair of monozygotic twins was included in an early epidemiology study,[2] and both the women developed HS in the breast region at the beginning of their third decade.

Case series evidence suggests that just more than one-third of patients with HS have a family history of the condition, one of the largest HS case series of 618 French patients reporting another affected family member in 35% of patients.[3] This figure, which relies on patient self-reporting, is probably an underestimate because family members may not discuss the condition between themselves because of embarrassment.

AUTOSOMAL DOMINANT INHERITANCE

The timeline of advances in the understanding of the genetics of HS (**Fig. 1**) begins in 1968 when Knaysi and colleagues[4] noted a family history of HS in 3 of 18 patients who were asked this question, in a case series of patients receiving surgical treatment of HS. Fitzsimmons and colleagues[2] took up the story in 1984, publishing a preliminary report of 3 UK families, including a total of 21 members with HS. All 3 generations of one family were affected. A year later, the same researchers expanded the study to include 23 families with a

Disclosure statement: The author has nothing to disclose.

Department of Dermatology & Wound Healing, University Hospital of Wales, Cardiff University, 3rd Floor Glamorgan House, Heath Park, Cardiff CF14 4XN, UK
E-mail address: ingramjr@cardiff.ac.uk

Dermatol Clin 34 (2016) 23–28
http://dx.doi.org/10.1016/j.det.2015.07.002
0733-8635/16/$ – see front matter

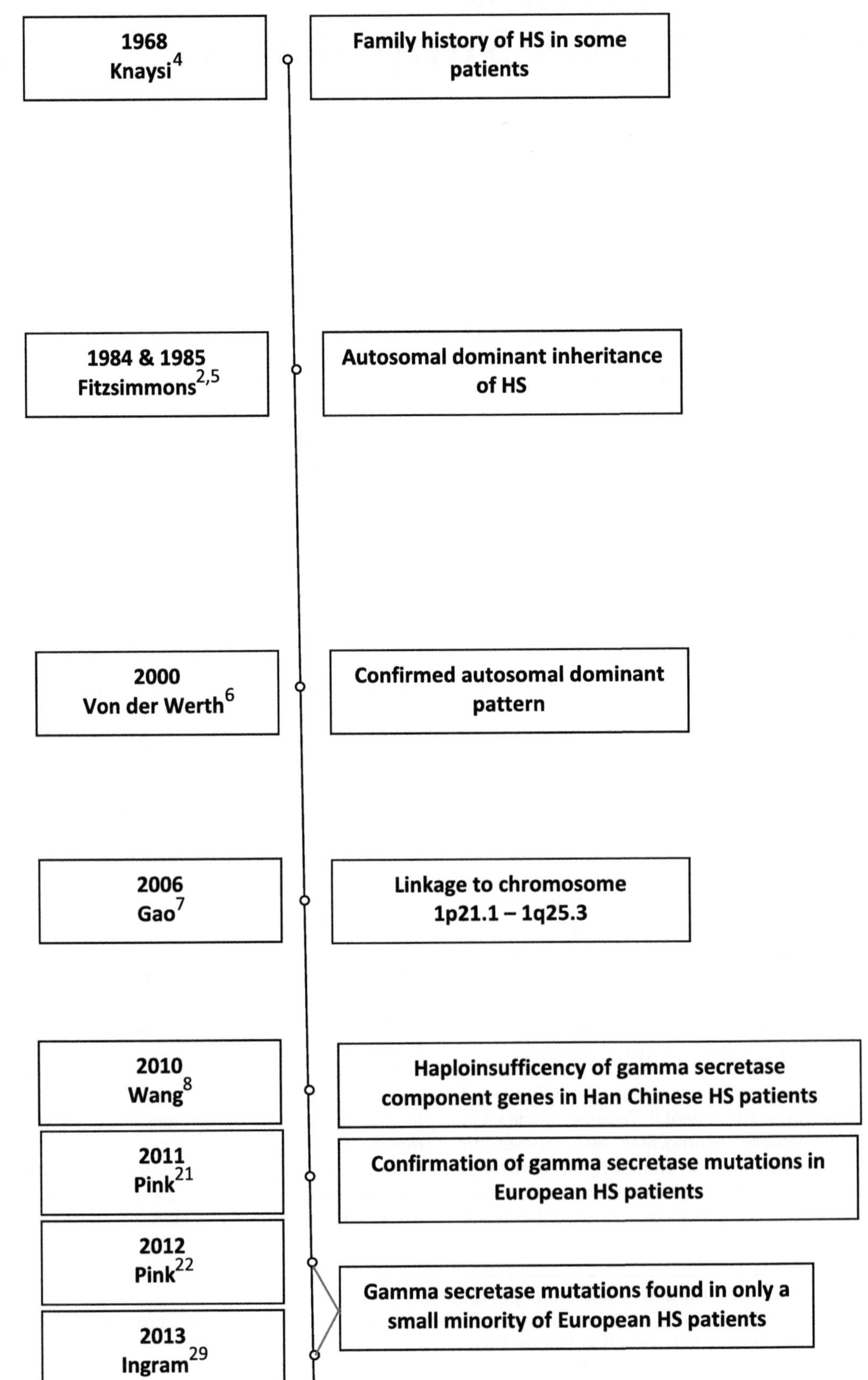

Fig. 1. Timeline of advances in the understanding of the genetics of hidradenitis suppurativa.

total of 62 affected individuals.[5] The disease definition used by the study was "recurrent suppurative cicatrizing lesions of apocrine gland bearing areas of the skin, primarily affecting the axillae and anogenital area." Vertical disease transmission was found involving all 3 generations in 5 families and 2 consecutive generations in 6 families, including male-to-male transmission. The researchers concluded that the pattern of inheritance suggested a single gene disorder inherited as an autosomal dominant trait.

For an autosomal dominant condition, the frequency of affected first-degree relatives should be 50%; however, in the Fitzsimmons study only 34% were affected.[5] The researchers argued that incomplete penetrance or incomplete case ascertainment may have contributed. In addition, younger unaffected relatives were included who could develop HS later in life, in the context that 16 of the 62 affected probands in the Fitzsimmons study did not develop HS until their fourth decade. In part to address this issue, Von der Werth and colleagues[6] reviewed 14 of the surviving probands in a subsequent study published in 2000. The researchers used a consensus disease definition involving a history of at least 5 painful, erythematous papules, nodules, or abscesses in the axillae or groins or at least 1 active lesion and a history of 3 others. Confirmed cases were individuals who conformed to the disease definition when assessed in person. Probable cases were those who met the definition when assessed by telephone but did not attend in person or individuals who had experienced several flexural skin boils but could not recall a sufficient number to meet the definition. Seven of the probands had a family history of HS, and of their 37 surviving first-degree relatives, 34 were included in the study. Of these, 10 individuals were confirmed to have HS, representing 27% of the total surviving first-degree relatives and including 2 people who had developed HS since the earlier study. Nine probable cases were also identified, producing a potential combined figure for affected first-degree relatives of 51%, with the caveat that about half did not entirely meet the disease definition.

LINKAGE TO CHROMOSOME 1

Building on the concept that susceptibility to HS may be underpinned by mutation in a single gene, Gao and colleagues[7] performed a whole-genome scan of individuals in a large Han Chinese family exhibiting autosomal dominant inheritance of HS across 4 generations. A clinical disease definition was used involving "inflammatory papules, painful nodules, pustules, sinuses and abscesses"; affected skin sites included the buttocks, axillae, scalp, face, neck, trunk, and limbs, and disease onset was between 10 and 20 years of age. A total of 9 affected family members and 6 unaffected members older than 10 years contributed to the linkage analysis. The genome-wide scan was performed using 382 fluorescent microsatellite markers and demonstrated linkage to chromosome 1. Subsequently, segregation between affected and unaffected family members of a further 20 microsatellite markers spanning the relevant portion of chromosome 1 was used to narrow down the genetic locus to a 73-Mb region containing approximately 886 genes, 1p21.1–1q25.3.

DISCOVERY OF γ-SECRETASE MUTATIONS IN HIDRADENITIS SUPPURATIVA

The combination of a genome-wide linkage scan and subsequent haplotype analysis described earlier was repeated by Wang and colleagues[8] in a further 6 Han Chinese families demonstrating autosomal dominant HS inheritance. Affected family members had skin lesions in both flexural and nonflexural skin sites, and the proband of family 1 also had a squamous cell carcinoma (SCC) of the left axilla. Linkage to chromosome 19q13 was found in families 1 and 2, and haplotype analysis narrowed the target to a 5.5 Mb region containing approximately 200 genes. Sequence analysis of candidate genes demonstrated a frameshift mutation in the *PSENEN* gene in affected members of family 1, a mutation that was absent in unaffected family members and 200 unrelated Han Chinese control individuals. *PSENEN* encodes 1 subunit of the γ-secretase protein. A different *PSENEN* frameshift mutation was present in affected members of family 2. In families 3 to 6, there was no *PSENEN* mutation, but sequence analysis revealed mutations in either *NCSTN* or *PSEN1*, genes that encode other γ-secretase subunits. The *NCSTN* gene is located at 1q22–23, within the region identified by Gao and colleagues.[7] Familial HS (acne inversa) is now listed in the Online Mendelian Inheritance in Man catalog under reference 142690 for *NCSTN* mutations, 613736 for *PSENEN* mutations, and 613737 for *PSEN1* mutations.

γ-SECRETASE STRUCTURE

The γ-secretase complex is composed of 4 different protein subunits, each with at least 1 transmembrane component. One of each subunit is required in the assembly of the functional protein, an intramembranous protease. The 4 subunits, presenilin, presenilin enhancer-2, nicastrin, and anterior pharynx defective, are encoded by a total of 6 genes, *PSEN1/PSEN 2, PSENEN, NCSTN*, and *APH1A/APH1B*, respectively. Presenilin is the proteolytic subunit and is itself activated by endoproteolysis by presenilin enhancer-2.[9] Nicastrin is required for maturation and stabilization of the protein complex,[10] and it may be that anterior pharynx defective also contributes to overall stability of the complex.

γ-SECRETASE FUNCTION

γ-Secretase is a protease the targets of which are type-1 transmembrane proteins such as amyloid precursor protein, Notch receptors, and members of the cadherin family. It has been extensively investigated because of PSEN1 and PSEN2 mutations being identified in familial Alzheimer disease,[11] which is characterized by an accumulation of β-amyloid peptides generated by cleavage of amyloid precursor protein. However, to date, an association between HS and familial Alzheimer disease has not been reported, despite neither being a rare condition. In addition, the γ-secretase mutations found in familial Alzheimer disease are nearly all missense, whereas the mutations in HS are mainly nonsense, frameshift, and splice site mutations expected to reduce protein function as a result of haploinsufficiency.[12,13]

The function of γ-secretase in human skin has been indirectly indicated by a γ-secretase inhibitor, semagacestat, which recently underwent an unsuccessful phase 3 trial for treatment of Alzheimer disease.[14] There was an increase in squamous cell and basal cell skin cancers, and hair and eyelash hypopigmentation was noted. In mouse models, γ-secretase deficiency results in conversion of hair follicles to epidermal cysts and absence of sebaceous glands,[15] the latter observation in keeping with a reduction in sebaceous gland volume and number in uninvolved hair follicles in humans with HS.[16] Nicastrin-deficient mice (*NCT* +/−) exhibit follicular and cystic hyperkeratosis, particularly in sebaceous gland–bearing regions of the skin.[17]

Mouse models have suggested that many of the effects of γ-secretase deficiency are mediated via the Notch signaling pathway. Notch 1–4 are cell membrane signaling receptors that can be activated by 5 ligands on neighboring cells, namely, Jagged1, Jagged2, or 3 Delta-like proteins.[18] Signal transduction requires γ-secretase proteolytic cleavage of the Notch intracellular domain, which then enters the nucleus to form a complex with C-promoter binding factor-1, a transcription factor,[19] affecting expression of genes involved in epidermal cell and hair follicle differentiation and proliferation.[20] Mice deficient in Notch 1, 2, and 3 exhibit skin changes similar to those that have a γ-secretase deficiency, in keeping with signal transduction via the γ-secretase Notch pathway.[15]

γ-SECRETASE MUTATIONS: TYPES AND GEOGRAPHIC LOCATIONS

Following the initial reports of γ-secretase mutations in Han Chinese families with HS, further γ-secretase mutations have been reported in patients with HS worldwide, including reports from the United Kingdom,[21,22] France,[23] and Japan[24] and in an African American family from the United States.[25] The reports continue to confirm that heterozygous mutations in *NCSTN, PSENEN*, and *PSEN1* are found in individuals with HS and most mutations are expected to produce haploinsufficiency of γ-secretase, potentially impairing Notch signaling. However, 4 of the reported γ-secretase mutations are missense *NCT* mutations,[22,26,27] and a recent study has provided evidence that these mutations do not impair Notch 1 signaling.[28]

ARE γ-SECRETASE MUTATIONS NECESSARY AND SUFFICIENT TO CAUSE HIDRADENITIS SUPPURATIVA?

The multiple reports of γ-secretase mutations in patients with HS in the literature give the impression that these may account for all cases of HS, particularly in those individuals with familial HS. However, a study that sequentially recruited 48 patients with HS attending a tertiary referral clinic, including 19 with a family history consistent with autosomal dominant inheritance, found γ-secretase mutations in only a minority of individuals.[22] Sequencing of *NCSTN, PSENEN*, and *PSEN1* demonstrated mutations in 3 individuals, although only 2 of the mutations were thought to be pathogenic. Neither of the 2 patients with pathogenic mutations reported a family history of HS, so no *NCSTN, PSENEN*, or *PSEN1* mutations were found in the 19 individuals exhibiting autosomal dominant inheritance. A further UK study found no pathogenic mutations on sequencing *PSEN1, PSEN 2, PSENEN, NCSTN, APH1A*, and *APH1B* in a series of 20 secondary care patients with HS, 12 of whom had a family history of HS in at least 1 first-degree relative.[29] These findings suggest that γ-secretase mutations underpin only a minority of cases of HS, even in those individuals with a positive family history.

A recent Japanese study has also suggested that a pathogenic γ-secretase mutation may be insufficient to produce the HS phenotype.[30] A nonsense *NCSTN* mutation was identified in 1 individual with HS, and this mutation was present in his brother, who also has HS, while being absent from nearly all unaffected family members and 100 ethnically matched control individuals. However, the *NCSTN* mutation was also present in the proband's 70-year-old sister who had no evidence of current HS on clinical examination and no history of HS in her lifetime. Unlike previous HS studies in multiplex kindreds, lack of complete cosegregation of a pathogenic γ-secretase mutation with the HS phenotype suggests that penetrance of the trait is less than 100%, leading to asymptomatic carriage of the mutation in this particular individual.

GENOTYPE-PHENOTYPE CORRELATIONS

Evidence is growing that, within the HS diagnostic category characterized by recurrent painful skin boils in flexural sites, there is a degree of heterogeneity producing a spectrum of disease. Canoui-Poitrine and colleagues[3] identified 3 possible subcategories of HS using latent class analysis, and the phenotype of patients with HS reported to have γ-secretase mutations fits best within their LC2 subcategory.[31] This group of patients, typified by the phenotype of the Han Chinese patients in whom γ-secretase mutations were first reported,[8] is characterized by involvement of nonflexural sites such as the back and chest, producing a degree of overlap or association with acne conglobata. Patients with γ-secretase mutations may have a more severe HS phenotype that is resistant to treatment.[22] Several cases of transformation to SCC have been noted in patients with HS with γ-secretase mutations,[8,30] which would fit with evidence that defects in Notch signaling may be involved in generation of cutaneous SCC.[32] However, the risk of SCC relative to patients with HS without γ-secretase mutations has not yet been determined.

FUTURE STUDIES

The disparity between a positive family history reported by at least one-third of patients with HS and the low rate of γ-secretase mutations suggests that other relevant genes await discovery. In particular, genes encoding other peptides involved in the Notch signaling pathway represent good candidates to investigate. Further work to accurately determine the phenotype of patients is also needed to improve genotype-phenotype correlations. Data are lacking regarding whether γ-secretase mutations alter the age of onset of HS relative to those without mutations and to accurately compare overall disease severity between mutation-positive and mutation-negative individuals. In addition, further data are needed regarding the effect of risk factors such as smoking and obesity on any genetic predisposition. Ultimately, the aim is to better understand the pathogenic pathways in HS, leading to more effective therapies for this disabling condition.

REFERENCES

1. Ingram JR, Abbott R, Ghazavi M, et al. The hidradenitis suppurativa priority setting partnership. Br J Dermatol 2014;171:1422–7.
2. Fitzsimmons JS, Fitzsimmons EM, Gilbert G. Familial hidradenitis suppurativa: evidence in favour of single gene transmission. J Med Genet 1984;21:281–5.
3. Canoui-Poitrine F, Le Thuaut A, Revuz JE, et al. Identification of three hidradenitis suppurativa phenotypes: latent class analysis of a cross-sectional study. J Invest Dermatol 2013;133:1506–11.
4. Knaysi GA Jr, Cosman B, Crikelair GF. Hidradenitis suppurativa. JAMA 1968;203:19–22.
5. Fitzsimmons JS, Guilbert PR, Fitzsimmons EM. Evidence of genetic factors in hidradenitis suppurativa. Br J Dermatol 1985;113:1–8.
6. Von der Werth JM, Williams HC, Raeburn JA. The clinical genetics of hidradenitis suppurativa revisited. Br J Dermatol 2000;142:947–53.
7. Gao M, Wang PG, Cui Y, et al. Inversa acne (hidradenitis suppurativa): a case report and identification of the locus at chromosome 1p21.1-1q25.3. J Invest Dermatol 2006;126:1302–6.
8. Wang B, Yang W, Wen W, et al. Gamma-secretase gene mutations in familial acne inversa. Science 2010;330:1065.
9. Kim SH, Sisodia SS. A sequence within the first transmembrane domain of PEN-2 is critical for PEN-2-mediated endoproteolysis of presenilin 1. J Biol Chem 2005;280:1992–2001.
10. Chavez-Gutierrez L, Tolia A, Maes E, et al. Glu(332) in the Nicastrin ectodomain is essential for gamma-secretase complex maturation but not for its activity. J Biol Chem 2008;283:20096–105.
11. Alzheimer's Disease Collaborative Group. The structure of the presenilin 1 (S182) gene and identification of six novel mutations in early onset AD families. Nat Genet 1995;11:219–22.
12. Pink AE, Simpson MA, Desai N, et al. γ-Secretase mutations in hidradenitis suppurativa: new insights into disease pathogenesis. J Invest Dermatol 2013;133:601–7.
13. Kelleher RJ 3rd, Shen J. Genetics. γ-secretase and human disease. Science 2010;330:1055–6.
14. Doody RS, Raman R, Farlow M, et al. A phase 3 trial of semagacestat for treatment of Alzheimer's disease. N Engl J Med 2013;369:341–50.

15. Pan Y, Lin MH, Tian X, et al. Gamma-secretase functions through Notch signaling to maintain skin appendages but is not required for their patterning or initial morphogenesis. Dev Cell 2004;7:731–43.
16. Kamp S, Fiehn AM, Stenderup K, et al. Hidradenitis suppurativa: a disease of the absent sebaceous gland? Sebaceous gland number and volume are significantly reduced in uninvolved hair follicles from patients with hidradenitis suppurativa. Br J Dermatol 2011;164:1017–22.
17. Li T, Wen H, Brayton C, et al. Epidermal growth factor receptor and notch pathways participate in the tumor suppressor function of gamma-secretase. J Biol Chem 2007;282:32264–73.
18. Melnik BC, Plewig G. Impaired Notch-MKP-1 signalling in hidradenitis suppurativa: an approach to pathogenesis by evidence from translational biology. Exp Dermatol 2013;22:172–7.
19. Fortini ME. Notch signaling: the core pathway and its posttranslational regulation. Dev Cell 2009;16:633–47.
20. Kwon SM, Alev C, Lee SH, et al. The molecular basis of Notch signaling: a brief overview. Adv Exp Med Biol 2012;727:1–14.
21. Pink AE, Simpson MA, Brice GW, et al. PSENEN and NCSTN mutations in familial hidradenitis suppurativa (acne inversa). J Invest Dermatol 2011;131:1568–70.
22. Pink AE, Simpson MA, Desai N, et al. Mutations in the γ-secretase genes NCSTN, PSENEN, and PSEN1 underlie rare forms of hidradenitis suppurativa (acne inversa). J Invest Dermatol 2012;132:2459–61.
23. Miskinyte S, Nassif A, Merabtene F, et al. Nicastrin mutations in French families with hidradenitis suppurativa. J Invest Dermatol 2012;132:1728–30.
24. Nomura Y, Nomura T, Sakai K, et al. A novel splice site mutation in NCSTN underlies a Japanese family with hidradenitis suppurativa. Br J Dermatol 2013;168:206–9.
25. Chen S, Mattei P, You J, et al. γ-Secretase mutation in an African American family with hidradenitis suppurativa. JAMA Dermatol 2015;151(6):668–70.
26. Li CR, Jiang MJ, Shen DB, et al. Two novel mutations of the nicastrin gene in Chinese patients with acne inversa. Br J Dermatol 2011;165:415–8.
27. Zhang C, Wang L, Chen L, et al. Two novel mutations of the NCSTN gene in Chinese familial acne inverse. J Eur Acad Dermatol Venereol 2013;27:1571–4.
28. Zhang X, Sisodia SS. Acne inversa caused by missense mutations in NCSTN is not fully compatible with impairments in Notch signaling. J Invest Dermatol 2015;135:618–20.
29. Ingram JR, Wood M, John B, et al. Absence of pathogenic γ-secretase mutations in a South Wales cohort of familial and sporadic hidradenitis suppurativa (acne inversa). Br J Dermatol 2013;168:874–6.
30. Nomura Y, Nomura T, Suzuki S, et al. A novel NCSTN mutation alone may be insufficient for the development of familial hidradenitis suppurativa. J Dermatol Sci 2014;74:180–2.
31. Ingram JR, Piguet V. Phenotypic heterogeneity in hidradenitis suppurativa (acne inversa): classification is an essential step towards personalised therapy. J Invest Dermatol 2013;133:1453–6.
32. South AP, Purdie KJ, Watt SA. NOTCH1 mutations occur early during cutaneous squamous cell carcinogenesis. J Invest Dermatol 2014;134:2630–8.

The Microbiology of Hidradenitis Suppurativa

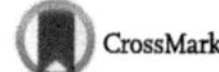

Hans Christian Ring, MD[a,*], Lennart Emtestam, MD[b]

KEYWORDS

• Hidradenitis suppurativa • Acne inversa • Microbiology • Bacteria • Colonization

KEY POINTS

- Coagulase-negative staphylococci (CoNS) and anaerobic bacteria are the most frequently isolated type of bacteria from patients with hidradenitis suppurativa (HS).
- Consistent findings of CoNS and *Corynebacterium* spp in deep tissue samples have been shown in HS.
- Biofilm formation has been found in HS lesions.
- Commensal bacteria may elicit inflammatory responses in genetically susceptible individuals.

INTRODUCTION

Although an increasing body of literature points to dysfunctional immune responses playing a key role in hidradenitis suppurativa (HS), involving both the innate and adaptive immune systems, the role of the microbiology remains in dispute. However, the clinical presentation is strongly reminiscent of bacterial infection and patients are often treated with antibiotics (eg, penicillins or incision) and drainage by nondermatologists, even though the treatments are regularly ineffective.

Whether bacterial colonization is a primary or secondary event in the evolution of HS lesions is a subject of much debate. In acne vulgaris a well-established correlation between disease development and *Propionibacterium acnes* are described.[1] No such clear association between a specific bacterium and the pathophysiology of HS has been shown. The literature on HS and its potential association with bacteria may seem bewildering, which may be attributed to the lack of consistency in methodology and different bacteriologic findings. Nevertheless, several studies have isolated an array of bacterial specimens sporadically associated with lesional HS tissue.[2–5] Consistent findings of gram-positive cocci and rods, including *Staphylococcus aureus*, coagulase-negative staphylococci (CoNS) and *Corynebacterium* spp in deep tissue samples have been shown in HS.[4,6] Although they are a part of the normal human skin flora they have been speculated to constitute a central target for the immune system in patients with HS. Moreover, the efficacy of antibiotics (ie, rifampicin, clindamycin, or tetracycline) in HS treatment further supports a microbial role in disease pathogenesis.[7,8] However, these antibiotics also work as immunomodulators, especially of T cells,[7,8] and the underlying mechanisms may therefore be more complex.

NORMAL BACTERIAL FLORA OF THE SKIN

A vast variety of microorganisms such as bacteria, fungi, and arthropods colonize the human skin. About 1 trillion commensal bacteria exist on the human skin surface, with Actinobacteria, Proteobacteria, Firmicutes, and Bacteroidetes as the overall dominant phyla.[9] The skin supports the

[a] Department of Dermatology, Roskilde Hospital, University of Copenhagen, Køgevej 7-13, Roskilde 4000, Denmark; [b] Department of Dermatology & Venereology, Karolinska University Hospital, Stockholm, Sweden
* Corresponding author.
E-mail address: hrin@regionsjaelland.dk

Dermatol Clin 34 (2016) 29–35
http://dx.doi.org/10.1016/j.det.2015.08.010
0733-8635/16/$ – see front matter

growth of commensal bacteria, which serves as an essential defense mechanism against pathogenic bacteria both directly and indirectly. For bacteria to become pathogenic they must possess specific properties, such as the ability to adhere, grow, and invade the host.[10] If organisms succeed in evading the cutaneous host defenses, the next line of protection involves the immune system, or skin-associated lymphoid tissue. However, the human skin is, in general, an unfavorable environment for bacterial growth because of the predominant dry areas on the skin surface.

An important feature of the skin is the topographic diversity of the bacterial populations, which depends on temperature, age, the amount of sebum, sweat production, hormonal status, and local humidity. Further, differentially distributed hair follicles, eccrine glands, apocrine glands, and sebaceous glands contribute to the variable cutaneous microenvironments, and are likely selective for the subsets of bacteria that can thrive in those specialized conditions.[9,11] The sites affected in HS (intertriginous areas) offer preferable conditions for bacterial growth because of their high levels of local humidity, sebaceous glands, sweat, and hair follicles.[12]

THE SPECTRUM OF BACTERIA FOUND IN PATIENTS WITH HIDRADENITIS SUPPURATIVA

Fig. 1 shows that CoNS (34.1%) and anaerobic bacteria (23.3%) were the most frequently encountered types of bacteria among the 324 patients included from 9 studies (see **Fig. 1**, **Table 1**). With regard to the overall categorization of the bacteria, facultative anaerobic bacteria constitute the highest percentage (69.6%) followed by strictly anaerobic bacteria (18.1%) and strictly aerobic bacteria (8.5%), whereas a less significant number of species were ungroupable (3.4%).

As seen in **Fig. 1**, the studies show a high prevalence of CoNS/coagulase positive staphylococci CoPS with a considerable variety of other species isolated from the inflamed lesions of patients with HS. Although there is no consistency with regard to the occurrence of the type of bacteria, all studies show predominantly positive culturing samples from HS lesions. The polymicrobial flora, and in particular the dominating occurrence of *S aureus*/CoNS in the HS lesions, may raise speculations on the pathogenetic significance of this recurring bacteriologic finding. However, although the microflora/microbiota of the normal human skin

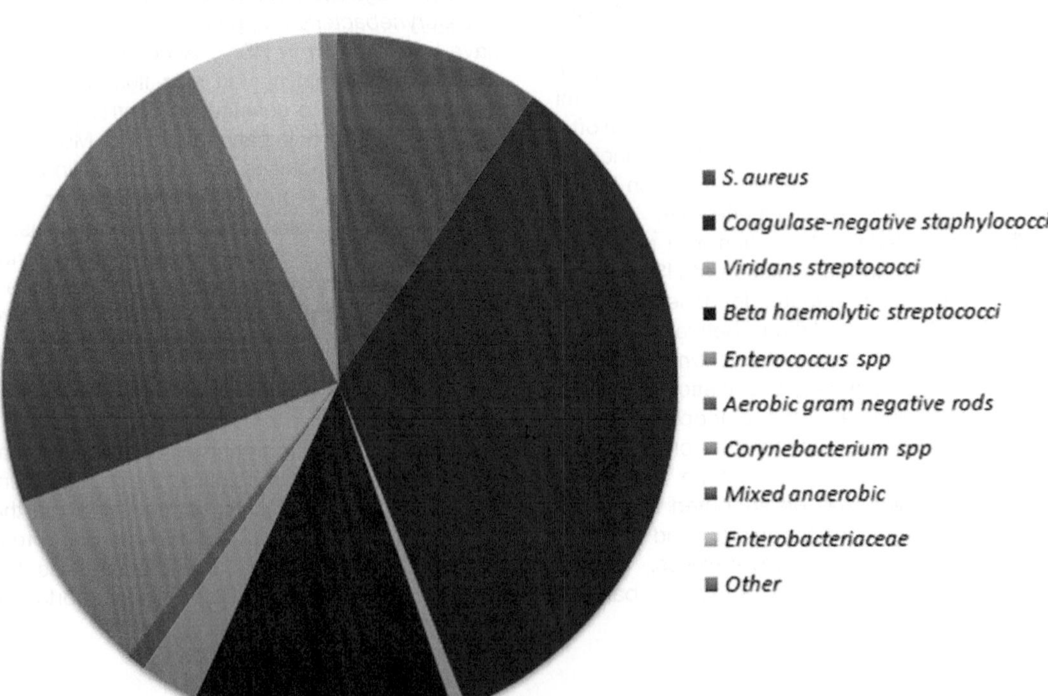

Fig. 1. Fractional distribution of various bacteria found in 9 studies. Swabs, biopsies, blood, and needle aspiration of purulent content are included. Bacteria that were not clearly identified as any of the bacteria listed earlier were not included in this presentation; for example, anaerobe streptococci, microaerophilic streptococci, anaerobe gram-positive cocci, and lactobacillus are classified as Other.

Table 1
Sampling methods of the studies and the most important bacteria found in HS lesions

Studies	Sampling Methods	Most Important Bacteria Found	Number of Patients Included (n)
Lapins et al,[6] 1999	Collection of tissue using CO_2	*S aureus* and CoNS	25
Matusiak et al,[3] 2014	Collection of pus after pressure of the lesion	CoNS, *Proteus mirabilis*, *S aureus*	69
Guet-Revillet et al,[5] 2014	Transcutaneous samples (punch biopsies and needle aspirations) and swabs	*Staphylococcus lugdunensis*, mixed anaerobic flora (strict anaerobes, *Streptococcus milleri* group and *Actinomyces* spp)	82
Highet et al,[42] 1988	Swabs of local discharge	*S milleri* group, *S aureus*, anaerobic streptococci	32
Sartorius et al,[4] 2012	Punch biopsies at 2 levels. Deep and superficial	CoNS, *Corynebacterium* spp	10
Brook & Frazier,[13] 1999	Needle aspiration of purulent contents	*S aureus*, *Streptococcus pyogenes*, *Peptostreptococcus* spp, *Bacteroides* spp	17
Sartorius et al,[23] 2006 [a]	Blood samples (8.3 mL)	CoNS, *P acnes*, *Propionibacterium granulosum*	21
Jemec et al,[14] 1996	Needle aspiration of purulent contents	*S aureus*, *S milleri* group, *Staphylococcus epidermidis*, *Staphylococcus hominis*	41
O'Loughlin et al,[43] 1988	Not applicable	*S epidermidis*, *S pyogenes*, anaerobic streptococci	27

[a] This study cultured strictly blood samples from patients with HS.

has been described,[11] no studies investigating the bacteriology in HS have included a healthy control group, which makes unequivocal conclusions on the possible pathogenic role of *S aureus* and CoNS, and the general polymicrobial flora, difficult. Moreover, subtyping of CoNS/CoPS is generally lacking. Nevertheless, a causal involvement of bacteria seems reasonable to many physicians, because the disease often responds to antibiotics and also has a clinical picture that resembles well-known colonization of wounds (suppuration).

STAPHYLOCOCCUS AUREUS

Although there is limited knowledge of the pathogenic properties of *S aureus* it is perhaps the most studied cutaneous pathogen. Nevertheless *S aureus* has often been described in association with HS and has even been proposed as a potential causative organism.[6,13,14] The bacterium is a facultative, gram-positive coccus known for its disease-causing capabilities (eg, food poisoning, skin infections, osteomyelitis, and endocarditis).[15] The specimen has been associated with well-established risk factors of HS, such as smoking.[16] Matusiak and colleagues[3] found that all their subjects with positive cultures of *S aureus* were heavy smokers. It has been speculated that an association between *S aureus* and nicotine may influence the disease development because nicotine may promote the growth of this pathogen.[17] Alternatively, Jemec and colleagues[14] proposed that *S aureus* may take part only in the initial process of disease development; for example, facilitating anatomic alterations in the hair follicles by inflammatory processes and necrosis.

Although colonization of *S aureus* is frequently encountered in other skin diseases (eg, atopic dermatitis and psoriasis vulgaris),[18,19] the clinical picture differs significantly compared with HS. It has often been stated that patients with from folliculitis decalvans (FD) express hypersensitivity to *S aureus*.[20] In FD, *S aureus* and a deficient host immune response seem to play an important role in development of this suppurative and cicatricial alopecia. A similar pathogenetic correlation may hypothetically be found in HS.

COAGULASE-NEGATIVE STAPHYLOCOCCI

The role of CoNS in the pathogenesis of HS is a frequently discussed topic in the literature. Several pathophysiologic theories involving CoNS bacteria are often speculated; for example, a combination of defects in the innate follicular immunity and overreactions to CoNS.[21]

Although the lesional evolution of HS may resemble CoNS infections (a slow and subacute evolutions), the clinical significance of CoNS, such as *Staphylococcus epidermidis*, is unclear, because they generally are considered to be nonpathogenic and a part of the normal skin flora.[10] Although CoNS are commensals of the skin and the mucosa they are known to cause severe infections in immune-suppressed patients.[22] The high occurrence of CoNS detected in previous studies may be explained by accidental contamination during the process of obtaining or culturing biopsies from the lesions. However, Lapins and colleagues[6] attempted to reduce this potential source of error by evaporate (using CO_2 laser ablation) the diseased tissue from the surface downwards, allowing sampling of bacteriologic cultures from the deep parts of the dermis, thereby reducing contamination with bacteria from superficial levels. Out of 25 patients with HS, Lapins and colleagues[6] found CoNS in 21 patients and 16 of these isolates were from deep levels of the skin. In addition, in 9 of the 16 deep samples, CoNS were the only bacteria detected, suggesting that commensals may represent an activating factor for the noninfectious inflammatory process in HS. This perspective raises the question of when and how a commensal becomes a pathogen. Although consistent results were shown in a similar but smaller study,[4] the significance of these findings may be questioned, because the same group of authors showed preoperative bacteremia in 9 of 21 patients with HS,[23] suggesting a continuous presence of bacteria in the blood. Moreover, the study showed that 15 of 29 staphylococci isolates were *Staphylococcus warneri*, which is normally part of the human skin but has also been considered a pathogen that may cause morbidity and mortality in hospitalized patients.[24]

A comprehensive study on the microbiology of 102 HS lesions from 82 patients using prolonged bacterial cultures and bacterial metagenomics found *Staphylococcus lugdunensis* in 58% of HS nodules and abscesses.[5] Strikingly, this specimen was associated with Hurley stage 1, which indicates a potential role in disease pathogenesis.

S lugdunensis may cause severe infections that are similar to those caused by *S aureus*, particularly acute endocarditis in prosthetic and native valves.[25,26] *S lugdunensis* has previously been reported as an important cause in skin and soft tissue infections, primarily in the pelvic girdle area.[27] Although it is normally known to colonize the areas below the waist, studies have pointed to a broader distribution of infected sites than is currently recognized. In a population-based epidemiologic study of patients infected with *S lugdunensis*, areas that possess apocrine sweat glands were the most frequently infected areas.[28] Thus it may be speculated that *S lugdunensis* belongs to the spectrum of commensal bacteria in areas that are also often affected in HS, namely the axillae, anogenital regions, and inframammary areas.

BIOFILM

Aggregates of bacteria encased in self-producing extracellular matrix material, the so-called biofilms, are often found in chronic wounds, and may inhibit the wound healing process.[29] An array of bacteria are capable of producing this extracellular matrix, which serves as a protective layer against host defense mechanisms and antimicrobial agents.[30] Biofilm infections are in general characterized by their recalcitrance to antibiotics and ability to circumvent host immune-mediated clearance, causing persistent infections.[31]

Chronic wounds are prone to secondary infection by bacteria because of loss of the innate, protective barrier function of the skin. HS lesions may seem consistent with the nature of chronic wounds because of their possible cause by endogenous mechanisms and failure to heal, or tendency to heal slowly, in an unpredictable manner.[32,33]

CoNS (and particularly *S epidermidis*) is notable for its propensity to form biofilms primarily associated with indwelling properties (eg, catheters and prostheses).[34] Biofilm configuration is the defining virulence factor associated with *S epidermidis*. Because *S epidermidis* has been isolated from superficial and deeper levels from HS nodules, HS may be capable of producing biofilm. Although the results are scarce, biofilm formation in HS has previously been described.[2,35] A histologic retrospective study of 27 patients with HS was performed using fluorescence in situ hybridization and immunofluorescence.[2] Biofilmlike structures were seen in one-fifth of the samples and were primarily situated in hair follicles and sinus tracts. In addition, it seems possible that chronic HS lesions resemble an environment such as that produced by a foreign body. One early inflammatory event in HS is a rupture of the follicular epithelium, followed by spilling of foreign body material, including corneocytes, bacteria, and hair, into the dermis. These products may initiate an inflammatory response that causes a foreign body granuloma. Epithelial strands induce the formation of sinuses in this inflammatory tissue. Secondary bacterial colonization may increase the chronic inflammation.[36] As previously described, CoNS are most often associated with hospital-acquired infections occurring on intravascular catheters[28] and prosthetic devices,[37] in which the presence of a foreign body enhances the pathogenic properties of CoNS. Therefore, it is tempting to believe that the milieu in HS can provide a comparable situation and thus enhance the pathogenic properties of CoNS. Further, sinus tracts in HS may also be ideal places for biofilm formation and this microbiologic principle may be applicable to CoNS in HS.

METHODS USED FOR BACTERIOLOGIC ANALYSIS

Studies attempting to analyze bacteria from HS lesions mainly rely on culture-based methods (see **Table 1**). About 1 trillion commensal bacteria exist on the human skin surface and, until recently, knowledge of the skin microbiota was primarily based on culture assays.[10] Although culture-based techniques have provided important insight into bacterial, fungal, and viral populations on the skin, the method is only able to culture less than 1% of the bacterial species present.[38] Moreover, culture-based methods exclude microbes that rely on microbe-microbe interactions to thrive.

Recent advances in culture-independent approaches using next-generation DNA sequencing offer researchers and clinicians new perspectives on the skin microbiome that are less biased than culture-based techniques.[39] Thus it seems attractive to investigate the microbiome of HS using a 16S ribosomal RNA gene approach. Regions within this gene give information on species-specific signature sequences, thereby providing useful data for bacterial identification. As seen in **Table 1**, only 1 HS study applied metagenomics. Although the study only performed metagenomics on 6 samples (swabs), it has paved the way for future research on bacteriology using metagenomics in case control studies. Such studies have already been performed on acne vulgaris,[1] psoriasis vulgaris,[19] and rosacea,[40] yielding major disease-associated findings.

Furthermore, with regard to the bacteriologic studies investigating the microflora in HS lesions, selection bias may be present, and generalization to patients with HS in the general population should be made with caution because studies have exclusively recruited patients with HS from the hospital population (ie, outpatient clinics or inpatients during HS operations). In addition, publication bias cannot be ruled out (ie, unpublished studies showing negative cultures).

SUMMARY

Although an array of studies has attempted to identify the role of bacteria in HS it is still evident that bacterial population structure and diversity at strain level is poorly understood in patients with HS. Because no uniform pattern of microflora in HS was observed in the previous pathobiological studies, the role of the residential microflora versus pathogens remains unknown. However, several promising theories involving bacteria have been proposed; for example, the hypothesis of commensal bacteria eliciting an inflammatory response in a genetically susceptible individual, causing keratin plugging of the hair follicle's infundibulum.[41]

The recurring findings of skin commensals in the deeper layers of HS point to potential causal mechanisms of disease development. Prospective studies providing insight on the skin microbiome at the strain level and genome level of particular dominant commensals in HS lesions may offer important knowledge in defining the role of bacteria in the pathogenesis of HS.

REFERENCES

1. Fitz-Gibbon S, Tomida S, Chiu BH, et al. *Propionibacterium acnes* strain populations in the human skin microbiome associated with acne. J Invest Dermatol 2013;133(9):2152–60.
2. Jahns AC, Killasli H, Nosek D, et al. Microbiology of hidradenitis suppurativa (acne inversa): a histological study of 27 patients. APMIS 2014;122(9):804–9.
3. Matusiak L, Bieniek A, Szepietowski JC. Bacteriology of hidradenitis suppurativa - which antibiotics are the treatment of choice? Acta Derm Venereol 2014;94(6):699–702.
4. Sartorius K, Killasli H, Oprica C, et al. Bacteriology of hidradenitis suppurativa exacerbations and deep tissue cultures obtained during carbon dioxide laser treatment. Br J Dermatol 2012;166(4):879–83.
5. Guet-Revillet H, Coignard-Biehler H, Jais JP, et al. Bacterial pathogens associated with hidradenitis suppurativa, France. Emerg Infect Dis 2014;20(12): 1990–8.

6. Lapins J, Jarstrand C, Emtestam L. Coagulase-negative staphylococci are the most common bacteria found in cultures from the deep portions of hidradenitis suppurativa lesions, as obtained by carbon dioxide laser surgery. Br J Dermatol 1999; 140(1):90–5.
7. Gener G, Canoui-Poitrine F, Revuz JE, et al. Combination therapy with clindamycin and rifampicin for hidradenitis suppurativa: a series of 116 consecutive patients. Dermatology 2009;219(2): 148–54.
8. van der Zee HH, Boer J, Prens EP, et al. The effect of combined treatment with oral clindamycin and oral rifampicin in patients with hidradenitis suppurativa. Dermatology 2009;219(2):143–7.
9. Hannigan GD, Grice EA. Microbial ecology of the skin in the era of metagenomics and molecular microbiology. Cold Spring Harb Perspect Med 2013;3(12):a015362.
10. Grice EA, Kong HH, Renaud G, et al. A diversity profile of the human skin microbiota. Genome Res 2008; 18(7):1043–50.
11. Human Microbiome Project Consortium. Structure, function and diversity of the healthy human microbiome. Nature 2012;486(7402):207–14.
12. Jemec GB. Clinical practice. Hidradenitis suppurativa. N Engl J Med 2012;366(2):158–64.
13. Brook I, Frazier EH. Aerobic and anaerobic microbiology of axillary hidradenitis suppurativa. J Med Microbiol 1999;48(1):103–5.
14. Jemec GB, Faber M, Gutschik E, et al. The bacteriology of hidradenitis suppurativa. Dermatology 1996;193(3):203–6.
15. Larkin EA, Carman RJ, Krakauer T, et al. *Staphylococcus aureus*: the toxic presence of a pathogen extraordinaire. Curr Med Chem 2009; 16(30):4003–19.
16. Kromann CB, Deckers IE, Esmann S, et al. Risk factors, clinical course and long-term prognosis in hidradenitis suppurativa: a cross-sectional study. Br J Dermatol 2014;171(4):819–24.
17. Kurzen H, Kurokawa I, Jemec GB, et al. What causes hidradenitis suppurativa? Exp Dermatol 2008;17(5):455–6.
18. Salah LA, Faergemann J. A retrospective analysis of skin bacterial colonisation, susceptibility and resistance in atopic dermatitis and impetigo patients. Acta Derm Venereol 2015;95(5):532–5.
19. Alekseyenko AV, Perez-Perez GI, De SA, et al. Community differentiation of the cutaneous microbiota in psoriasis. Microbiome 2013;1(1):31.
20. Otberg N, Kang H, Alzolibani AA, et al. Folliculitis decalvans. Dermatol Ther 2008;21(4):238–44.
21. Scheinfeld N. Hidradenitis suppurativa: a practical review of possible medical treatments based on over 350 hidradenitis patients. Dermatol Online J 2013;19(4):1.
22. von EC, Peters G, Heilmann C. Pathogenesis of infections due to coagulase-negative staphylococci. Lancet Infect Dis 2002;2(11):677–85.
23. Sartorius K, Lapins J, Jalal S, et al. Bacteraemia in patients with hidradenitis suppurativa undergoing carbon dioxide laser surgery: detection and quantification of bacteria by lysis-filtration. Dermatology 2006;213(4):305–12.
24. Kamath U, Singer C, Isenberg HD. Clinical significance of *Staphylococcus warneri* bacteremia. J Clin Microbiol 1992;30(2):261–4.
25. Jones RM, Jackson MA, Ong C, et al. Endocarditis caused by *Staphylococcus lugdunensis*. Pediatr Infect Dis J 2002;21(3):265–8.
26. Patel R, Piper KE, Rouse MS, et al. Frequency of isolation of *Staphylococcus lugdunensis* among staphylococcal isolates causing endocarditis: a 20-year experience. J Clin Microbiol 2000;38(11): 4262–3.
27. Bellamy R, Barkham T. *Staphylococcus lugdunensis* infection sites: predominance of abscesses in the pelvic girdle region. Clin Infect Dis 2002;35(3): E32–4.
28. Bocher S, Tonning B, Skov RL, et al. *Staphylococcus lugdunensis*, a common cause of skin and soft tissue infections in the community. J Clin Microbiol 2009;47(4):946–50.
29. Bjarnsholt T, Kirketerp-Moller K, Jensen PO, et al. Why chronic wounds will not heal: a novel hypothesis. Wound Repair Regen 2008;16(1):2–10.
30. Costerton JW, Lewandowski Z, Caldwell DE, et al. Microbial biofilms. Annu Rev Microbiol 1995;49: 711–45.
31. Namvar AE, Bastarahang S, Abbasi N, et al. Clinical characteristics of *Staphylococcus epidermidis*: a systematic review. GMS Hyg Infect Control 2014; 9(3):Doc23.
32. Bowler PG. Wound pathophysiology, infection and therapeutic options. Ann Med 2002;34(6):419–27.
33. Schultz GS, Sibbald RG, Falanga V, et al. Wound bed preparation: a systematic approach to wound management. Wound Repair Regen 2003;11(Suppl 1):S1–28.
34. Fey PD, Olson ME. Current concepts in biofilm formation of *Staphylococcus epidermidis*. Future Microbiol 2010;5(6):917–33.
35. Kathju S, Lasko LA, Stoodley P. Considering hidradenitis suppurativa as a bacterial biofilm disease. FEMS Immunol Med Microbiol 2012;65(2): 385–9.
36. Plewig G, Kligman AM. Acne inversa. In: Acne and rosacea. 2nd edition. New York: Springer-Verlag; 1993.
37. Dougherty SH. Pathobiology of infection in prosthetic devices. Rev Infect Dis 1988;10(6):1102–17.
38. Grice EA. The skin microbiome: potential for novel diagnostic and therapeutic approaches to

cutaneous disease. Semin Cutan Med Surg 2014; 33(2):98–103.

39. Buchan BW, Ledeboer NA. Emerging technologies for the clinical microbiology laboratory. Clin Microbiol Rev 2014;27(4):783–822.
40. Casas C, Paul C, Lahfa M, et al. Quantification of *Demodex folliculorum* by PCR in rosacea and its relationship to skin innate immune activation. Exp Dermatol 2012;21(12):906–10.
41. van der Zee HH, Laman JD, Boer J, et al. Hidradenitis suppurativa: viewpoint on clinical phenotyping, pathogenesis and novel treatments. Exp Dermatol 2012;21(10):735–9.
42. Highet AS, Warren RE, Weekes AJ. Bacteriology and antibiotic treatment of perineal suppurative hidradenitis. Arch Dermatol 1988; 124(7):1047–51.
43. O'Loughlin S, Woods R, Kirke PN, et al. Hidradenitis suppurativa. Glucose tolerance, clinical, microbiologic, and immunologic features and HLA frequencies in 27 patients. Arch Dermatol 1988; 124(7):1043–6.

The Role of Mechanical Stress in Hidradenitis Suppurativa

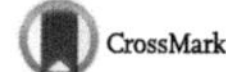

Jurr Boer, MD, PhD[a,*], Maiwand Nazary, MSc[b], Peter Theut Riis, MD[c]

KEYWORDS

- Hidradenitis suppurativa • Acne inversa • Mechanical stress • Friction • Follicular disease
- Pilonidal sinus • Acne mechanica • Limb amputees

KEY POINTS

- Mechanical stress can act as a possible trigger in the development of hidradenitis suppurativa (HS).
- The role of mechanical stress has been supported by the special biomechanical conditions in the typically topographic areas of HS and the indirect proof of similar findings in associated follicular occlusion diseases such as acne mechanica and pilonidal sinus disease, and in limb amputees after expression of mechanical forces.
- Support of mechanical stress has also substantiated by pathohistologic, ultrasonography, and immunologic findings.
- Overweight patients seem to be most susceptible to the effects of mechanical stress.

INTRODUCTION

Hidradenitis suppurativa (HS) is a chronic, painful, and inflammatory skin disorder of unknown origin, affecting inverse skin areas and associated with a high burden of disease.[1–3] The diagnosis is made clinically, based on the patients' history of recurrent typical lesions such as tender subcutaneous nodules or abscesses and tunnels (sinus tracts[4]) in the prototypical areas. HS was originally thought to be a disease of the apocrine sweat glands. However, more recent data indicate that HS is a disease originating from the hair follicles, following follicular occlusion by infundibular hyperkeratinization and dilatation of the follicle with subsequent rupture, which are thought to be the first events in HS.[5–8]

There are conflicting reports about the influence of external physical or chemical factors on the development of HS. Patients claim that their condition deteriorates as a result of external factors, ranging from sweating to shaving.[9] An association has been shown between shaving the affected areas before the onset of HS and earlier disease onset.[10] However, a retrospective study showed that factors such as deodorants, depilatory products, and shaving did not influence HS in a negative manner.[11] Hitherto, no experimental evidence has been shown in support of mechanical stress as a cause of HS. In contrast, in a questionnaire-based survey, it was shown that tight clothing or friction aggravated patients' HS and that they obtained some relief when avoiding tight-fitting clothes.[9] The role of mechanical stress is also supported by 3 case reports and 1 pathology study that suggested increased fragility of the dermoepidermal junction, which suggest that mechanical stress may contribute or be causative in the development of HS.[12–16] Additional observations also suggest that an interplay may exist between

[a] Department of Dermatology, Deventer Hospital, N. Bolkesteinlaan 75, Deventer 7416 SE, The Netherlands; [b] Division of Pharmacology, Utrecht Institute for Pharmaceutical Sciences, University of Utrecht, PO Box 80.082 Utrecht 3508 TB, The Netherlands; [c] Department of Dermatology, Roskilde Hospital, Kogevej 7-13, Roskilde DK-4000, Denmark
* Corresponding author.
E-mail address: jurrboer@home.nl

Dermatol Clin 34 (2016) 37–43
http://dx.doi.org/10.1016/j.det.2015.08.011

mechanical stress on the epidermis and the development of HS lesions.

MECHANICAL STRESS OF THE SKIN

There are various kinds of mechanical stress: pressure, friction, shearing forces, stretching, rubbing, tension, pulling, pinching, and almost all other types of physical forces that act on the skin. Tribological (friction/rubbing science) studies have helped clinicians to understand the role of friction as a causative agent in various dermatologic events. Friction or frictional force, which may be defined as the resistance to motion in a direction relative to the common boundary of 2 surfaces, is a significant mechanical force that can cause tissue ischemia resulting in skin breakdown.[17] There is a substantial difference between frictional forces and shear forces, or sheer stress, which is defined as force per unit area exerted parallel to the plane of interest.[18] Sheer injury is not observed at the skin level because it occurs in deeper skin layers. A common example of shear force is when a person sitting in a wheelchair slides forward while the skin on the buttocks adheres to the surface of the seat cushion. This type of motion can result in pressure sores or decubitus ulcers, which are usually seen in persons confined to bed for long periods of time.[19] In contrast, friction may occur on tight dressings, skin-to-skin contact (as seen in obese individuals), and continuous frictional skin contact with external material. Body areas at greatest risk for such frictional forces are largely the axillae, groins, buttocks, neck, and waistline.[20] **Table 1** lists the effects of the different kinds of mechanical stress.

Table 1
Effects of the different types of mechanical stress

Type of Mechanical Stress	Presentation	Layers of Skin Affected
Pressure	Pressure ulcers	Epidermis, dermis, subcutis
Friction	Friction blister, intertrigo, lichenification, HS, acne mechanica	Epidermis
Shearing	Pressure ulcers	Subcutis, dermis
Stretching and tension	Lichenification	Epidermis

ETIOPATHOPHYSIOLOGY

The primary events in HS are follicular plugging (infundibulo)folliculitis, and dilatation of the follicle. In predisposed subjects, such a folliculitis can develop to the more serious and extended HS stages, classically in the inverse skin areas, a hallmark of HS. The question arises: why does this involvement happen in the regions with this typical topography? Pathohistologic studies have shown that within these affected regions the follicles are always involved.[21] Moreover, the inflammation starts deep in the follicle around the bulbus, and continuous laterally.[5,22] Furthermore, investigations using ultrasonography to visualize HS lesions showed abnormalities in the hair follicles of the axillae and groins.[23,24] A consistent finding was the widened hair follicles in the affected areas, indicating enlargement and distortion of the base of the hair follicle in early stages. In more advanced stages, dermal and subcutaneous tracts were found, commonly connected to the base of the hair follicles. The widening of the follicles seems to represent an anatomic predisposition rather than a reactive pattern to existing disease.[24] A child was recently described who developed HS-like lesions in an inguinal nevus comedonicus following increased mechanical stress on the region. The patient had a biopsy-verified congenital skin abnormality characterized by dilated hair follicles grouped in the inguinal fold. It had also been speculated that mechanical stress applied to follicles of a given size or width may provoke HS.[12] However, in a later study, Kamp and colleagues[25] failed to find any indication of increased follicular diameter in HS samples.

The biomechanical circumstances of the inverse or concave skin areas are different from those of convex skin regions.[26] The anatomy and properties of the skin show differences. It has been observed, by means of sonographic investigations, that an abnormal dermal thickening is present in the axillary and genitofemoral regions, while the axillary skin is thinner than in the genitofemoral region. It was postulated that the increased dermal thickness, resulting in alterations of the mechanical conditions of the inverse skin areas, could be the physical factor in the development of HS. However, it remains to be shown whether the skin thickening is a primary manifestation in HS or the result of chronic inflammation.[24] The special biomechanical circumstances are also supported by histologic findings of the normal axillary skin, which showed a ruffled surface as opposed to convex body sites such as the face. Moreover, the epidermal surface of the axillary skin affected by HS is thrown into folds.[27] It has been postulated that constant mechanical forces, such as friction in the axillae and groins, contributes to microcomedo formation, considered an early step in the cascade of development of HS, which may lead to infrafollicular hyperkeratinization, dilatation of the follicle, and eventually microtears and rupture of the follicle wall with ensuing abscesses.[26,27] This process is enhanced by obesity (discussed later).[26,28] It has also been suggested that microtears of the hair follicle of predisposed subjects may even be the primary event.[26] It has been postulated that HS may be caused by defective follicular support. The sebofollicular junction in HS skin was found to be a thinning of the periodic acid schiff (PAS)-positive material along the basement membrane zone, which may explain the apparent fragility of this junction. It may be hypothesized that, in individuals with such a predisposition, exposure to mechanical stress easily leads to damaged and subsequently ruptured follicles.[14] These biomechanical mechanisms in the affected areas are stimulated in particular in the obese. It is widely accepted that obesity is a risk factor for HS and it is indicated that there is a dose-response effect with a positive correlation between disease severity and degree of body mass index.[29,30] Moreover, it has been found that weight loss can ameliorate disease symptoms.[15,31,32] There are several explanations why obesity may aggravate or contribute to the development of HS. The skin-to-skin contact is intensified in the intertriginous locations, especially in the deep skin folds. These folds could be the abdominal folds but also the axillae of obese patients, in whom the axillae are between the enlarged lateral thoracic walls and the upper arms, resulting in overlapping skin folds and subsequently an increase of maceration and friction.[3,33] Mechanical stress in such obese patients contributes to the retention of the hair follicle material (ie, corneocytes, hair shafts, sweat, and sebaceous products), leading to plugging of the follicle opening, follicle dilation, and the whole cascade of the development of HS.[26] Moreover, in these skin folds, a warm, humid, occlusive microclimate develops, favoring microbial growth.[13,28] Furthermore, the fat mass by itself is associated with a low-grade systemic inflammatory state, capable of producing adipokines, cytokines, and chemokines.[28,34,35] Recently, an obese patient with classic HS was described who developed HS lesions in the abdominal skin folds as well as on the upper abdomen, at the height of the waistband. This finding suggests that not only the low-grade inflammatory state of the fat mass but also the mechanical stress may be a contributing factor in the development of HS.[15] In that case, unspecific factors such as mechanical stress or friction might initiate the inflammation. It would be useful to know whether mechanical stretching or friction of the skin has an effect on the keratinocytes, and, if so, how this event is translated by the epidermal keratinocytes. Mechanical stress induces the proliferation of epidermal keratinocytes under influence of calcium signaling.[36] Moreover, this induction is further increased by the presence of ATP.[37] Mechanical stress also strongly increases the release of the proinflammatory enzyme matrix metalloproteinase 9 in human keratinocytes.[38] Furthermore, mechanical stress is also responsible for the thickening of the epidermis (hyperplasia) and hyperkeratosis through an increase of keratinocyte differentiation and proliferation after the mechanical stimuli.[39] Recent studies of wound repair models show that fibroblast but not keratinocytes secrete the epidermal growth factor responsible for keratinocyte migration in wound healing.[40]

Some genes related to wound healing are downregulated in keratinocytes as a response to mechanical stress. The downregulation is on a messenger RNA level and has been shown in skin grown from human embryonic stem cells. The genes are connexin 43, laminin α5, interleukin α, endothelin 1, and keratinocyte growth factor.[41] The fact that mechanical stress may induce cell proliferation, while suppressing genes related to wound healing, underlines that keratinocyte responses to mechanical forces are still poorly understood.

THE ROLE OF MECHANICAL STRESS IN HIDRADENITIS SUPPURATIVA–ASSOCIATED FOLLICULAR DISEASES

HS has been associated with follicular occlusion disorders such as acne conglobata, dissecting cellulitis of the scalp (DC), and pilonidal sinus (acne tetrad). A patient may have 2 or more conditions within the tetrad. The most commonly linked disorders are HS and acne conglobata, closely followed by HS and pilonidal sinus. The association between HS and DC is rare.[42,43] Although some studies report a strong association between HS and acne vulgaris, which could increase up to 70%, other studies have shown that the linkage with acne vulgaris is not increased.[3,42]

A variant is acne mechanica, whereby acne lesions develop at locations exposed to mechanical stress in acne-prone patients.[44] Although the existence of acne or acnelike eruption is not necessary to diagnose this, mechanical stress is, necessary in order to make the diagnosis.[45] Mills and Kligman[44] described experimental induction of crops of inflammatory lesions, such as pustules, papules, and even nodules, in patients with moderate to severe acne, after being subjected to moderate levels of mechanical stress. No comedones were induced by physical forces. A similar (inflamed) acne eruption with cysts was found on the necks of concert violinists under the poorly fitting chin rest of their violins.[46] Headbands and helmets worn by athletes are other causes of similar lesions compatible with early HS. Pathohistologic examination showed plugged, dilated hair follicles with a high degree of perilesional inflammation.[44,45] The different presentations of acne mechanica are presented in **Table 2**.

Pilonidal sinus disease (PSD) is a disease of the upper natal cleft or sacrococcygeal area that can develop by mechanical stress and pressure in the presence of hair.[47] The cause of PSD has been controversial. Initially the cause was thought to be congenital, whereas it is now widely considered an acquired disorder. Evidence for this includes[1] that PSD does not occur at birth but occurs mainly at a young age, and[2] that PSD is well known for its association with military personnel. It was called Jeep's disease because this condition was widespread in the United States Army during the Second World War; most of the army personnel who were being hospitalized rode in jeeps, traveling on rough ground, which caused friction, pressure, and shearing forces.[48] PSD may affect other anatomic areas as well, such as the beard, the belly button, and the web spaces of the hand (Barber's hand), which are anatomic regions generally exposed to high levels of frictional forces.[49,50] It was hypothesized that the hair follicles in these regions became distended, filled with keratin, and then ruptured[51] Recently it was suggested in 2 pathology studies that PSD is caused by keratin plugs and debris[52] and that PSD and HS have common characteristics at the histologic and immunologic levels.[53] Furthermore, studies using ultrasonography showed a constituent finding of abnormal structural connections of fluid collections and fistulous tracts with the base of hair follicles, as well as in HS as PSD.[54] These findings indicate that HS and PSD are related diseases in which mechanical stress plays a significant role.

Table 2
Examples of acne mechanica

Examples of Acne Mechanica	Localization
Fiddler's neck	On left side off the neck, just below the jaw
Turtle-neck shirt and sweater acne	Neck
Stump acne	Amputation stump, pressure areas from prosthetics
Acne keloidalis nuchae	Regio nuchae on American football players
Sweat band	Forehead

A variant of the follicular occlusion triad has been described in a patient in a vegetative state who also had classic HS in the genital area. The patient developed HS-like lesions on his chin. Initially, recurrent inflammatory pustules and papules developed on his chin, which was attributed to a change of shaving the patient (ie, a blade was replaced by an electric razor). The razor was used aggressively and often caused redness and even bleeding over the chin. After daily, aggressive, and traumatic shaving for years with an electric razor, these lesions developed into deep-seated pustules and inflammatory nodules, progressively increasing in size on the chin and behind the ears, eventually resulting in abscessed and fibrotic masses on the chin. Histology of early lesions showed follicular plugging and an infundibulofolliculitis, compatible with HS.[7,55]

These 3 examples of follicular occlusion diseases (acne mechanica, PSD, and HS-like lesions on the chin) show morphologically and pathologically similar features to HS after expression of mechanical stress. In all 3 disorders there were similar histologic features of the early, initial lesions; namely follicular hyperkeratosis or plugging, followed by distension and eventually bursting of the follicle.

THE ROLE OF MECHANICAL STRESS IN LIMB AMPUTEES

Limb amputees present with several mechanical diseases of the skin. The use of prostheses may induce skin disorders, such as acroangiodermatitis, allergic contact dermatitis, infections, ulcerations, and epidermal hyperplasia, including epidermoid cysts, verrucous hyperplasia, hyperkeratotic papules, and acne mechanica.[56] Most of these skin problems have a mechanical and a nonmechanical part in their development. In particular, friction, shear forces, and pressure may contribute to the onset of contact dermatitis, epidermal hyperplasia, and ulcerations.[56] In 2 older studies, the appearance of multiple cysts, commonly called posttraumatic epidermoid cysts, in the groin were described in above-knee amputees. In the milder forms of the disorder, small keratin plugs were present in the groin region. With the ongoing process, deep, extremely tender cysts were seen. In severe cases, intercommunicating sinuses appeared in the groin, sometimes connected by firm cords. Fibrotic structures were described, which contained sinuses with fluid discharge. Bacterial studies of the fluid showed mainly sterile pus. Pathohistologic studies of the early stages showed follicular plugging. In more advanced cases, cysts and sinus tracts with epidermal walls were found in the dermis. Both the cysts and the sinus tracts contained keratin. The diagnosis of HS was not made by the investigators.[57,58]

However, the findings fit perfectly with HS. As seen in these 2 reports, limb amputees wearing prostheses seem (almost) a model for the development of HS by mechanical stress. It was recently hypothesized that mechanical stress is a risk factor for HS from a patient with a lower leg amputation who presented HS-like lesions on his leg stump after wearing a leg prosthesis. The investigators postulated that predilection sites of HS correspond with areas of mechanical friction, in combination with a warm, moisturized, occlusive microclimate favorable to bacteria.[13]

There is consensus that HS is an inflammatory disease in which several factors initiate a specific inflammatory cascade. It has been postulated that all of these different stimuli trigger an abnormal innate immune response and may lead to similar HS lesions. Beside bacterial, host defense, genetic, and endocrinologic factors, exogenous factors such as mechanical stress can also act as possible triggers. The role of mechanical stress has been supported by (1) the special biomechanical conditions in the typically topographical areas of HS, (2) the indirect proof of similar findings in associated follicular occlusion diseases such as acne mechanica, PSD and limb amputees after expression of mechanical forces, (3) it has been substantiated by pathohistological, ultrasound and immunological findings and finally, overweight patients appear to be most susceptible to the effects of mechanical stress.

REFERENCES

1. Revuz J. Hidradenitis suppurativa. J Eur Acad Dermatol Venereol 2009;23:985–98.
2. Jemec GB. Clinical practice: hidradenitis suppurativa. N Engl J Med 2012;366:158–64.
3. Alikhan A, Lynch PJ, Eisen DB. Hidradenitis suppurativa: a comprehensive review. J Am Acad Dermatol 2009;60:539–61.
4. Freysz M, Jemec GB, Lipsker D. A systematic review of terms used to describe hidradenitis suppurativa. Br J Dermatol 2015. [Epub ahead of print].
5. von Laffert M, Helmbold P, Wohlrab J, et al. Hidradenitis suppurativa (acne inversa): early inflammatory events at terminal follicles and at interfollicular epidermis. Exp Dermatol 2010;19:533–7.
6. Jemec GB, Hansen U. Histology of hidradenitis suppurativa. J Am Acad Dermatol 1996;34(6):994–9.
7. Boer J, Weltevreden EF. Hidradenitis suppurativa or acne inversa. A clinicopathological study of early lesions. Br J Dermatol 1996;135:721–5.
8. Jemec GB, Thomsen BM, Hansen U. The homogeneity of hidradenitis suppurativa lesions. A histological study of intra-individual variation. APMIS 1997; 105(5):378–83.
9. von der Werth JM, Williams HC. The natural history of hidradenitis suppurativa. J Eur Acad Dermatol Venereol 2000;14:389–92.
10. Matusiak L, Bieniek A, Szepietowski JC. Hidradenitis suppurativa and associated factors: still unsolved problems. J Am Acad Dermatol 2009;61:362–5.
11. Morgan WP, Leicester G. The role of depilation and deodorants in hidradenitis suppurativa. Arch Dermatol 1982;118:10.
12. Dufour DN, Bryld LE, Jemec GB. Hidradenitis suppurativa complicating naevus comedonicus: the possible influence of mechanical stress on the development of hidradenitis suppurativa. Dermatology 2010;220:323–5.
13. De Winter K, van der zee HH, Prens EP. Is mechanical stress an important pathogenic factor in hidradenitis suppurativa? Exp Dermatol 2012; 21:176–7.
14. Danby FW, Jemec GB, Marsch W Ch, et al. Preliminary findings suggest hidradenitis suppurativa may be due to defective follicular support. Br J Dermatol 2013;168:1034–9.
15. Boer J. Resolution of hidradenitis suppurativa after weight loss through dietary measures, with emphasis on locations exposed to mechanical stress. J Eur Acad Dermatol Venereol 2015. http://dx.doi.org/10.1111/jdv.13059.
16. Zouboulis CC, Desai N, Emtestam L, et al. European S1 guideline for the treatment of hidradenitis suppurativa/acne inversa. J Eur Acad Dermatol Venereol 2015;29(4):619–44.
17. An executive summary of the National Pressure Ulcer Advisory Board Panel monograph. Pressure ulcers in America: prevalence, incidence, and implications for the future. Adv Skin Wound Care 2012;14:208–15.
18. Gupta S, Baharestani M, Baranoski S, et al. Guidelines for management pressure ulcers with negative pressure wound therapy. Skin Wound Care 2004;17: 1–16.
19. Soban LM, Hempel S, Munjas BA, et al. Preventing pressure ulcers in hospitals: a systemic review of nurse-focused quality improvement interventions. Jt Comm J Qual Patient Saf 2011;37:24552.

20. Slade DE, Powell BW, Mortimer PS. Hidradenitis suppurativa: pathogenesis and management. Br J Plast Surg 2003;56:451–61.
21. Yu CW, Cook MG. Hidradenitis suppurativa: a disease of follicular epithelium rather than apocrine glands. Br J Dermatol 1990;122:763–9.
22. Von Laffert M, Stadie V, Wohlrab J, et al. Hidradenitis suppurativa/acne inversa: bilocated epithelial hyperplasia with very different sequelae. Br J Dermatol 2011;164:367–71.
23. Wortsman X, Jemec GB. Real-time imaging ultrasound of hidradenitis suppurativa. Dermatol Surg 2007;33:1340–2.
24. Jemec GB, Gniadecka M. Ultrasound examination of hair follicles in hidradenitis suppurativa. Arch Dermatol 1997;133:967–70.
25. Kamp S, Fiehn AM, Stenderup K, et al. Hidradenitis suppurativa: a disease of the absent sebaceous gland? Sebaceous gland number and volume are significantly reduced in uninvolved hair follicles from patients with hidradenitis suppurativa. Br J Dermatol 2011;164:1017–22.
26. Kurzen H, Kurakawa I, Jemec GB, et al. What causes hidradenitis suppurativa? Exp Dermatol 2008; 17:455–72.
27. Sellheyer K, Krahl D. "Hidradenitis suppurativa" is acne inversa! An appeal to (finally) abandon a misnomer. Int J Dermatol 2005;44:535–40.
28. Van der Zee HH, Laman JD, Boer J, et al. Hidradenitis suppurativa: a viewpoint on clinical phenotyping, pathogenesis and novel treatments. Exp Dermatol 2012;21:21735–9.
29. Sartorius K, Entestam L, Jemec GB, et al. Objective scoring of hidradenitis suppurativa reflecting the role of tobacco smoking and obesity. Br J Dermatol 2009;161:831–9.
30. Canoui-Poitrine F, Revuz JE, Wolkenstein P, et al. Clinical characteristics of a series of 302 French patients with hidradenitis suppurativa with an analysis of factors associated with disease severity. J Am Acad Dermatol 2009;61:51–7.
31. Thomas CL, Gordon KD, Mortimer PS. Rapid resolution of hidradenitis suppurativa after bariatric surgical intervention. Clin Exp Dermatol 2014;39: 315–8.
32. Kromann CB, Ibler KS, Kristianssen VB, et al. The influence of body weight on the prevalence and severity of hidradenitis suppurativa. Acta Derm Venereol 2014;94:533–7.
33. Edlich RF, Silloway KA, Rodeheaver GT, et al. Epidemiology, pathology, and treatment of axillary hidradenitis suppurativa. J Emerg Med 1986;4: 369–78.
34. Deckers IE, van der Zee HH, Prens EP. Epidemiology of hidradenitis suppurativa: prevalence, pathogenesis, and factors associated with the development of HS. Curr Derm Rep 2014;3:54–60.
35. Nazary M, van der Zee HH, Prens EP, et al. Pathogenesis and pharmacotherapy of hidradenitis suppurativa. Eur J Pharmacol 2011;672:1–8.
36. Yano S, Komine M, Fujimoto M, et al. Activation of Akt by mechanical stretching in human epidermal keratinocytes. Exp Dermatol 2006;15:356–61.
37. Tsutsumi M, Inoue K, Denda S, et al. Mechanical-stimulation-evoked calcium waves in proliferating and differentiated human keratinocytes. Cell Tissue Res 2009;338:99–106.
38. Reno F, Traina V, Cannas M. Mechanical stretching modulates growth direction and MMP-9 release in human keratinocyte monolayer. Cell Adh Migr 2009;3(3):239–42.
39. Ajani G, Sato N, Mack JA, et al. Cellular responses to disruption of the permeability barrier in a three-dimensional organotypic epidermal model. Exp Cell Res 2007;313:3005–15.
40. Lü D, Gao Y, Huo B, et al. Asymmetric migration of human keratinocytes under mechanical stretch and cocultured fibroblasts in a wound repair model. PLoS One 2013;8(9):e74563.
41. Cherbuin T, Movahednia MM, Toh WS, et al. Investigation of human embryonic stem cell-derived keratinocytes as an in vitro research model for mechanical stress dynamic response. Stem Cell Rev 2015;11(3): 460–73.
42. Fimmel S, Zouboulis CC. Comorbidities of hidradenitis suppurativa (acne inversa). Dermatoendocrinol 2010;1:9–16.
43. Scheinfeld NS. A case of dissecting cellulitis and a review of the literature. Dermatol Online J 2014;20:2.
44. Mills OH, Kligman MA. Acne mechanica. Arch Dermatol 1975;111:481–3.
45. Strauss RM, Harrington CI. Stump acne: a new variant of acne mechanica and a cause of immobility. Br J Dermatol 2001;144:628–50.
46. Peachy RD, Matthews CN. Fiddler's neck'. Br J Dermatol 1978;98:669–74.
47. Breuninger H. Treatment of pilonidal sinus and acne inversa. Hautarzt 2004;55(3):254–8.
48. Humphries AE, Duncan JE. Evaluation and management of pilonidal disease. Surg Clin North Am 2010; 90:113–24.
49. Efthimiadis C, Kosmidis C, Anthimidis G, et al. Barber's hair sinus in a female hairdresser: uncommon manifestation of an occupational disease: a case report. Case J 2008;1(1):214.
50. Sion-Vardy N, Osyntsov L, Cagnano E, et al. Unexpected location of pilonidal sinuses. Clin Exp Dermatol 2009;34:599–601.
51. Bascom J. Pilonidal disease: origin from follicles of hairs and results of follicle removal as treatment. Surgery 1980;87:567–72.
52. Søndenaa K, Pollard ML. Histology of chronic pilonidal sinus. APMIS 1995;103:267–72.

53. Von Laffert M, Stadie V, Ulrich J, et al. Morphology of pilonidal sinus disease: some evidence of its being a unilocalized type of hidradenitis suppurativa. Dermatology 2011;223:349–55.
54. Wortsman X, Moreno C, Soto R, et al. Ultrasound in-depth characterization and staging of hidradenitis suppurativa. Dermatol Surg 2013;39(12): 1835–42.
55. Meyers SW, Bercovitch L, Polley K, et al. Massive exophytic abscesses and fibrotic masses of the chin: a variant of the follicular occlusion tetrad. J Am Acad Dermatol 2003;48:S47–50.
56. Meulenbelt HE, Geertzen JH, Dijkstra PU, et al. Skin problems in lower limb amputees: an overview by case reports. J Eur Acad Dermatol Venereol 2007; 21:147–55.
57. Allende MF, Levy SW, Barnes GH. Epidermoid cysts in amputees. Acta Derm Venereol 1963;43:56–67.
58. Levy SW. Skin problems of the leg amputee. Prosthet Orthot Int 1980;4:37–44.

Endocrinologic Aspects of Hidradenitis Suppurativa

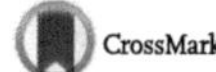

Ioannis Karagiannidis, MD[1], Georgios Nikolakis, MD, PhD[1], Christos C. Zouboulis, MD, PhD*

KEYWORDS

• Hidradenitis suppurativa • Acne inversa • Endocrinology • Androgens • Apocrine glands • Obesity • Metabolic syndrome • Hyperandrogenism

KEY POINTS

- Although the pathophysiology of hidradenitis suppurativa (HS) remains controversial, it is likely that endocrinologic factors play some role in its pathogenesis and maintenance.
- The exact association between sex hormones and occurrence of HS remains unclear.
- Despite normal androgen profiles in most patients, an abnormal peripheral conversion of androgens by the apocrine glands may induce a hormonal dysregulation in situ.
- Obesity is a well-known trigger factor of HS.
- Diabetes, dyslipidemia, polycystic ovarian syndrome, and thyroid disease are among the commonest comorbid disorders.

INTRODUCTION

The occurrence of hidradenitis suppurativa (HS) in a narrow age spectrum after puberty and predominantly in obese patients suggests that endocrinologic factors may be involved in the pathogenesis of HS. Although its pathophysiology is still not elucidated, HS, similar to acne, is a disease of follicular plugging and subsequent inflammation.[1,2] Based on this fact, endocrinologic disorders associated with follicular diseases could be proposed to be involved in the pathophysiologic pathway of HS. In a large, retrospective, case-control study including 2292 patients with HS, comorbid endocrinologic/metabolic disorders such as dyslipidemia, polycystic ovarian syndrome, diabetes, and thyroid disease were among the commonest group reported.[3,4]

HIDRADENITIS SUPPURATIVA AND SEX HORMONES

Association with acne vulgaris, irregular menses, hirsutism, and higher concentrations of total testosterone and free androgen index has been documented in a study.[5] Exacerbations of the disease have also been reported with menses.[1] Shorter menstrual cycles and longer duration of menstrual flow are correlated with the disease[6] and absence of a premenstrual flare of the disease is associated with anovulatory or irregular menstrual circles.[7] Decreased progesterone levels were documented in female patients without premenstrual flares.[7] Onset after menopause is rare.

Interestingly, further studies provided contradictory data: basal levels of major sex hormones, such as estrogens, progesterone, testosterone,

Departments of Dermatology, Venereology, Allergology and Immunology, Dessau Medical Center, Auenweg 38, 06847 Dessau, Germany
[1] The authors contributed equally to the study.
* Corresponding author.
E-mail address: christos.zouboulis@klinikum-dessau.de

Dermatol Clin 34 (2016) 45–49
http://dx.doi.org/10.1016/j.det.2015.08.005
0733-8635/16/$ – see front matter

dehydroepiandrosterone sulfate in serum were not found significantly altered in comparison to controls.[8] Moreover, signs of virilization are not common in HS patients.[2] A prospective study with 70 females with HS failed to show a significant difference in acne, hirsutism and irregular menstruation.[6]

Because the majority of HS patients exhibit normal androgen levels, it has been suggested that the pathophysiology of the disease correlates with an enhanced peripheral conversion of androgens,[9,10] introducing for the first time the idea of HS being a disease based on in situ hormonal dysregulation. However, the activity of three peripheral androgen-converting enzymes in apocrine glands of the axilla of HS patients showed no differences in comparison with those of the controls.[10] An interesting immunohistologic analysis from axillary, inguinal, and perianal skin biopsies deriving from 16 women and 8 men suffering from HS tried to provide evidence for a difference in apocrine gland androgen receptor and estrogen receptor expression. In accordance with previous findings, no alterations in androgen receptor or estrogen receptor expression were reported in biopsies deriving from lesional HS skin in comparison with controls.[11]

Increased free androgen levels may be a result of low levels of sexual hormone–binding globulin as reported in patients with increased body weight.[2,12] In these cases, an increased free androgen index does not necessarily indicate hyperandrogenism. Although the majority of HS patients have normal androgen profiles, there are reports of significant remission after antiandrogen therapy.[13–16] In a double-blinded study conducted by Mortimer and colleagues,[17] the antiandrogen cyproterone acetate (50 mg) in conjunction with ethinyl estradiol (50 μg) led to complete or partial clearance in 50% of 24 female patients after 18 months of treatment.[17] Kraft and Searles[13] studied retrospectively a case series of 64 female patients with HS. In this group of patients, the antiandrogen therapy was superior to oral antibiotic therapy (55% vs 26%), although the *P* value was marginal (<0.04). In contrast, the use of oral contraceptives containing progestogens may worsen the course of the disease or even induce it, because of their proandrogenic properties.[15] In the recently published S1 guideline for HS,[18] the use of oral contraceptives with antiandrogenic potential is suggested for female patients with menstrual abnormalities, signs of hyperandrogenism (seborrhea, acne, hirsutism, androgenetic alopecia syndrome[19,20]), and upper normal or increased serum levels of dehydroepiandrosterone, androstenedione and/or sexual hormone–binding globulin.

The antiandrogenic diuretic spironolactone was also reported to have beneficial results in the treatment of HS.[21] HS is rarely a feature of premature adrenarche, supporting the aspect of an androgen-dependent disorder.[22,23] Interestingly, the disease frequently improves during pregnancy.[2,24] Inhibitors of type II 5α-reductase can also be a therapeutic option in HS, especially in recalcitrant cases. Joseph and colleagues[25] used the type II 5α-reductase inhibitor finasteride (5 mg/d) in a pilot study with 7 patients, who did not respond well to antibiotic treatment. Six of the 7 patients showed a significant clinical improvement and 2 of the 6 showed complete remission of the lesions.

HIDRADENITIS SUPPURATIVA AND METABOLIC DISORDERS

HS is considered as one of the skin comorbid disorders of obesity.[4,26] It primarily affects obese women in the third to fourth decade,[27] about 3.3 times more often than men of the same age.[28–31] In 2 recent, large, cross-sectional studies including 3207 patients and 326 patients, there was a clear association between HS and the metabolic syndrome.[32,33] HS patients present almost all metabolic syndrome criteria, including hypertriglyceridemia, central obesity, hypo–high-density lipoprotein cholesterolemia, and hyperglycemia.[18,34] The clinical efficacy of metformin in treating cases of HS that have not responded to standard therapies supports further this association.[25] A retrospective chart review was conducted by Gold and colleagues[35] investigated the correlation of HS and the metabolic syndrome. This study, which included 366 patients with HS, showed a clear correlation of disease with the prevalence of the metabolic syndrome (50.6% in the HS group in comparison with only 30.2% in the control group).[35]

Metformin has been proposed as an effective HS treatment in patients who have not responded to standard therapies in case reports and in a clinical study.[16,36,37] In the clinical study, 25 patients were treated with metformin over a period of 24 weeks, and 18 clinically improved with a significant average reduction in their Sartorius score of 12.7 and number of monthly work days lost reduced from 1.5 to 0.4.[37] The Dermatology Life Quality Index also showed a significant improvement in 16 cases, with a decrease in the Dermatology Life Quality Index score of 7.6.

HIDRADENITIS SUPPURATIVA AND THE HYPOTHALAMUS–PITUITARY AXIS

A functional disorder of the hypothalamus pituitary axis was found in 13 patients with HS when compared with 9 controls. The results of combined thyrotropin-releasing hormone and gonadotropin-releasing hormone test conducted on HS patients and healthy controls reported that the prolactin and thyroid-stimulating hormone responses were significantly greater in the HS patients than in the controls.[8] HS has also been reported to be associated with endocrine disorders, such as Cushing syndrome[38] and acromegaly.[39]

HIDRADENITIS SUPPURATIVA AND THE HORMONAL MICROENVIROMENT

Apart from endocrinologic disorders documented in a macroscopic level, one should bear in mind the potential impairment(s) of in situ hormone production and metabolism in HS skin. There is extensive evidence that human skin and in particular skin annexes (sebaceous gland, hair follicle) are able to both produce de novo and metabolize a wide spectrum of peptide and steroid hormones.[40–45] Kamp and colleagues[46] determined the volume of sebaceous glands deriving from lesional skin of 21 patients with HS and compared it with that of 9 controls, and found the sebaceous gland volume reduced in HS. In some cases, a complete absence was reported.[46] Sebocytes express various enzymes, allowing the pathway to proceed with final production of glucocorticoids and sex hormones. Moreover, they possess the enzyme machinery to produce steroid hormones de novo from cholesterol.[47] Their unique ability to convert dehydroepiandrosterone to testosterone in situ and regulate their balance bidirectionally and the expression of all three isotypes of 5α-reductase underlines their dominant role in skin steroidogenesis.[43,48–50] From the data presented, it is clear that a disturbance in circulating androgen levels is not necessarily essential for hormone-related pathophysiologic alterations in skin homeostasis of HS patients. A dysregulation of hormonal balance in the periphery of target organs, such as the skin, may suffice to initiate the primary stages of the disease, such as follicular plugging as the result of hyperkeratinization. The reduction of sebaceous gland volume[46] provides a suggestion of a disturbance of the in situ hormonal homeostasis. Further studies are required to elucidate a potential hormonal dysregulation in HS skin.

SUMMARY

From these data, there are indications for an endocrinologic/metabolic contribution to HS pathogenesis. However, the existing data are not sufficient to include endocrinologic disorders as an independent factor of HS pathophysiology. Based on the currently available evidence, the endocrine changes seem more likely to be confounding factors resulting from hormonal fluctuations associated with the most significant risk factors, such as obesity. On the other hand, hormonal therapies (antiandrogens, metformin) comprise a therapeutic option for cases of recalcitrant HS or other comorbidities based on hormonal dysregulation.

REFERENCES

1. von der Werth JM, Williams HC. The natural history of hidradenitis suppurativa. J Eur Acad Dermatol Venereol 2000;14:389–92.
2. Revuz J. Hidradenitis suppurativa. J Eur Acad Dermatol Venereol 2009;23:985–98.
3. Shlyankevich J, Chen AJ, Kim GE, et al. Hidradenitis suppurativa is a systemic disease with substantial comorbidity burden: a chart-verified case-control analysis. J Am Acad Dermatol 2014;71:1144–50.
4. Miller IM, Holzman RJ, Hamzavi I. Prevalence, risk factors, and co-morbidities of HS. Derm Clin 2015, in press.
5. Mortimer PS, Dawber RP, Gales MA, et al. Mediation of hidradenitis suppurativa by androgens. Br Med J (Clin Res Ed) 1986;292:245–8.
6. Jemec GBE. The symptomatology of hidradenitis suppurativa in women. Br J Dermatol 1988;119: 345–50.
7. Harrison BJ, Read GF, Hughes LE. Endocrine basis for the clinical presentation of hidradenitis suppurativa. Br J Surg 1988;75:972–5.
8. Harrison BJ, Kumar S, Read GF, et al. Hidradenitis suppurativa: evidence for an endocrine abnormality. Br J Surg 1985;72:1002–4.
9. Kurzen H, Kurokawa I, Jemec GBE, et al. What causes hidradenitis suppurativa? Exp Dermatol 2008;17:455–6.
10. Barth JH, Kealey T. Androgen metabolism by isolated human axillary apocrine glands in hidradenitis suppurativa. Br J Dermatol 1991;125:304–8.
11. Buimer MG, Wobbes T, Klinkenbijl JHG, et al. Immunohistochemical analysis of steroid hormone receptors in hidradenitis suppurativa. Am J Dermatopathol 2015; 37:129–32.
12. Barth JH, Layton AM, Cunliffe WJ. Endocrine factors in pre- and postmenopausal women with hidradenitis suppurativa. Br J Dermatol 1996;134:1057–9.
13. Kraft JN, Searles GE. Hidradenitis suppurativa in 64 female patients: retrospective study comparing oral antibiotics and antiandrogen therapy. J Cutan Med Surg 2007;11:125–31.
14. Goldsmith PC, Dowd PM. Successful therapy of the follicular occlusion triad in a young woman with high dose oral antiandrogens and minocycline. J R Soc Med 1993;86:729–30.

15. Stellon AJ, Wakeling M. Hidradenitis suppurativa associated with use of oral contraceptives. BMJ 1989;298:28–9.
16. van der Zee HH, Gulliver W. Other medical treatments of hidradenitis suppurativa. Derm Clin 2015, in press.
17. Mortimer PS, Dawber RP, Gales MA, et al. A double-blind controlled cross-over trial of cyproterone acetate in females with hidradenitis suppurativa. Br J Dermatol 1986;115:263–8.
18. Zouboulis CC, Desai N, Emtestam L, et al. European S1 guideline for the treatment of hidradenitis suppurativa/acne inversa. J Eur Acad Dermatol Venereol 2015;29:619–44.
19. Orfanos CE, Adler YD, Zouboulis CC. The SAHA syndrome. Horm Res 2000;54:251–8.
20. Camacho FM. SAHA syndrome: female androgenetic alopecia and hirsutism. Exp Dermatol 1999;8: 304–5.
21. Salavastru CM, Fritz K, Tiplica GS. Spironolacton in dermatologischen Behandlungen. Hautarzt 2013; 64:762–7.
22. Lewis F, Messenger AG, Wales JKH. Hidradenitis suppurativa as a presenting feature of premature adrenarche. Br J Dermatol 1993;129:447–8.
23. Palmer RA, Keefe M. Early-onset hidradenitis suppurativa. Clin Exp Dermatol 2001;26:501–3.
24. Margesson LJ, Danby FW. Hidradenitis suppurativa. Best Pract Res Clin Obstet Gynaecol 2014; 28:1013–27.
25. Joseph MA, Jayaseelan E, Ganapathi B, et al. Hidradenitis suppurativa treated with finasteride. J Dermatolog Treat 2005;16:75–8.
26. Yosipovitch G, DeVore A, Dawn A. Obesity and the skin: skin physiology and skin manifestations of obesity. J Am Acad Dermatol 2007;56:901–20.
27. Meixner D, Schneider S, Krause M, et al. Acne inversa. J Dtsch Dermatol Ges 2008;6:189–96.
28. Schmitt JV, Bombonatto G, Martin M, et al. Risk factors for hidradenitis suppurativa: a pilot study. An Bras Dermatol 2012;87:936–8.
29. Jemec GB, Heidenheim M, Nielsen NH. The prevalence of hidradenitis suppurativa and its potential precursor lesions. J Am Acad Dermatol 1996;35: 191–4.
30. Revuz JE, Canoui-Poitrine F, Wolkenstein P, et al. Prevalence and factors associated with hidradenitis suppurativa: results from two case-control studies. J Am Acad Dermatol 2008;59:596–601.
31. Canoui-Poitrine F, Revuz JE, Wolkenstein P, et al. Clinical characteristics of a series of 302 French patients with hidradenitis suppurativa, with an analysis of factors associated with disease severity. J Am Acad Dermatol 2009;61:51–7.
32. Shalom G, Freud T, Harman-Boehm I, et al. Hidradenitis suppurativa and the metabolic syndrome. A comparative cross-sectional study of 3,207 patients. Br J Dermatol 2015. http://dx.doi.org/10.1111/bjd.13777.
33. Miller IM, Ellervik C, Vinding GR, et al. Association of metabolic syndrome and hidradenitis suppurativa. JAMA Dermatol 2014;150:1273–80.
34. Sabat R, Chanwangpong A, Schneider-Burrus S, et al. Increased prevalence of metabolic syndrome in patients with acne inversa. PLoS One 2012;7: e31810.
35. Gold DA, Reeder VJ, Mahan MG, et al. The prevalence of metabolic syndrome in patients with hidradenitis suppurativa. J Am Acad Dermatol 2014;70: 699–703.
36. Arun B, Loffeld A. Long-standing hidradenitis suppurativa treated effectively with metformin. Clin Exp Dermatol 2009;34:920–1.
37. Verdolini R, Clayton N, Smith A, et al. Metformin for the treatment of hidradenitis suppurativa: a little help along the way. J Eur Acad Dermatol Venereol 2013;27:1101–8.
38. Curtis AC. Cushing's syndrome and hidradenitis suppurativa. Arch Derm Syphilol 1950;62:329–30.
39. Chalmers RJ, Ead RD, Beck MH, et al. Acne vulgaris and hidradenitis suppurativa as presenting features of acromegaly. Br Med J (Clin Res Ed) 1983;287: 1346–7.
40. Slominski A, Zbytek B, Nikolakis G, et al. Steroidogenesis in the skin: implications for local immune functions. J Steroid Biochem Mol Biol 2013;137: 107–23.
41. Labrie F, Luu-The V, Labrie C, et al. Intracrinology and the skin. Horm Res 2000;54:218–29.
42. Paus R, Arck P, Tiede S. (Neuro-)endocrinology of epithelial hair follicle stem cells. Mol Cell Endocrinol 2008;288:38–51.
43. Zouboulis CC. Human skin: an independent peripheral endocrine organ. Horm Res 2000;54:230–42.
44. Zouboulis CC. The skin as an endocrine organ. Dermatoendocrinol 2009;1:250–2.
45. Zouboulis CC, Chen WC, Thornton MJ, et al. Sexual hormones in human skin. Horm Metab Res 2007;39: 85–95.
46. Kamp S, Fiehn AM, Stenderup K, et al. Hidradenitis suppurativa: a disease of the absent sebaceous gland? Sebaceous gland number and volume are significantly reduced in uninvolved hair follicles from patients with hidradenitis suppurativa. Br J Dermatol 2011;164:1017–22.
47. Thiboutot D, Jabara S, McAllister JM, et al. Human skin is a steroidogenic tissue: steroidogenic enzymes and cofactors are expressed in epidermis, normal sebocytes, and an immortalized sebocyte cell line (SEB-1). J Invest Dermatol 2003;120: 905–14.
48. Fritsch M, Orfanos CE, Zouboulis CC. Sebocytes are the key regulators of androgen homeostasis in human skin. J Invest Dermatol 2001;116:793–800.

49. Chen W, Thiboutot D, Zouboulis CC. Cutaneous androgen metabolism: basic research and clinical perspectives. J Invest Dermatol 2002;119: 992–1007.

50. Chen W, Tsai SJ, Sheu HM, et al. Testosterone synthesized in cultured human SZ95 sebocytes derives mainly from dehydroepiandrosterone. Exp Dermatol 2010;19:470–2.

Inflammatory Mechanisms in Hidradenitis Suppurativa

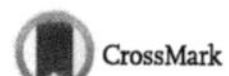

G. Kelly, MB, MRCPI[a,*], Errol P. Prens, MD, PhD[b]

KEYWORDS

• Hidradenitis suppurativa • Inflammation • Immunology • Pathogenesis • Cytokines

KEY POINTS

- Cytokines involved in hidradenitis suppurativa (HS) pathogenesis include interleukin (IL)-1β, IL-17, IL-10 and to a lesser extent TNF-α, therefore representing potential therapeutic targets.
- An overzealous toll-like receptor response to commensal bacteria may be an initiating factor in the the pathogenesis of this disease. In advanced stages, characterised by sinus tract formation and scarring, superinfection with bacterial strains known to induce soft tissue infection may occur, which frequently responds to intensive targeted antibiotic therapy.
- Smoking is epidemiologically linked to HS. The mechanism of action of smoking in initiating or propagating HS is theoretically by:
  - Inducing epidermal hyperplasia and keratinization, leading to occlusion of the follicular infundibulum
  - Alteration of the skin immune response
  - Increasing microbial virulence and decreasing skin antimicrobial peptides

INTRODUCTION

Hidradenitis suppurativa (HS) is a chronic, debilitating disease with significant associated psychosocial morbidity.[1] Reflecting the lack of an established pathogenic pathway, treatments for HS remain suboptimal.[2] A growing body of research and evidence, however, is paving the way for better management of patients with this difficult condition. The key to unlocking therapeutic options may be the elucidation of the inflammatory mechanisms at the core of the disease process.

Follicular occlusion, as opposed to apocrinitis, is central to the development of HS.[3] The cause of this is likely multifactorial. Environmental triggers (eg, cigarette smoking and adiposity) in a genetically susceptible individual result in the HS phenotype.[4,5] The role of aberrant immunity in HS has become topical and is suggested by an association with other immune-mediated diseases such as Crohn's disease and pyoderma gangrenosum, and by a favorable response to tumor necrosis factor alpha (TNF-α) blockade.[5] It is suggested that immune mechanisms contribute to follicular occlusion. This is hypothesized as innate and adaptive immune cells (and their products) are found in abundance in lesional and perilesional skin, and are thought to precede clinically apparent HS.[5,6] Despite scientific advancement, the exact pathogenic pathways are poorly defined, and the precise cytokine profile in HS has not been fully elucidated.[5]

Conflict of interest: None declared.

[a] Department of Dermatology, St. Vincent's University Hospital, Dublin 4, Ireland; [b] Department of Dermatology, Erasmus University Medical Centre Rotterdam, s-Gravendijkwal 230, 3015 CE Rotterdam, Netherlands
* Corresponding author.
E-mail address: gkellywinter@gmail.com

Dermatol Clin 34 (2016) 51–58
http://dx.doi.org/10.1016/j.det.2015.08.004
0733-8635/16/$ – see front matter

CYTOKINES IN HIDRADENITIS SUPPURATIVA

There is a lack of consensus as to which cytokines and immune pathways drive the inflammation in HS. TNF-α is a pivotal proinflammatory cytokine, produced by innate and adaptive immune cells, and it has an established role in many inflammatory conditions such as psoriasis, Crohn disease, rheumatoid arthritis, sarcoidosis, and uveitis.[7] Because clinical improvement in HS is frequently observed with infliximab[8] and adalimumab treatment,[9] it is hypothesized that TNF-α expression is enhanced in this disease. Several studies have demonstrated the presence of TNF-α at mRNA and protein levels in HS skin samples compared to healthy controls, and in some cases, comparable to levels in psoriatic skin.[6,10–13] Dréno and colleagues[14] found that the protein concentration of TNF-α was in fact decreased in lesional and perilesional HS skin compared with healthy controls, suggesting deficient cutaneous innate immunity. A limitation of this study however, is that conclusions were drawn based on immunohistochemical analysis using paraffin-embedded tissue sections only, which limit firm interpretation. Other studies looked at circulating concentrations of TNF-α in peripheral blood/serum, again with conflicting results. Giamarellos-Bourboulis and colleagues[15] demonstrated a diminished innate response to lipopolysaccharide stimulation in HS, with monocytes from patients producing less TNF-α than healthy controls. A possible explanation of these in vitro results may be that they are caused by in vivo anti-inflammatory priming of HS monocytes (eg, by the high interleukin [IL]-10 levels in HS). In contrast, Matusiak and colleagues[16] demonstrated enhanced concentrations of TNF-α in HS serum. In a study by van der Zee and colleagues[17] looking at the effects of adalimumab on cytokine expression in HS skin, biopsies were taken before and at week 16 after treatment. The protein expression of TNF-α and its receptors was enhanced in HS skin before treatment, but not as prominently as other cytokines such as IL-1β and IL-10 when compared with healthy control skin (1.6-fold increase vs 54 and 14.8 respectively). Similarly, the response to adalimumab was not as marked on TNF-α concentrations than these other cytokines. Another recent study demonstrated enhanced mRNA expression of TNF-α in lesional and perilesional HS skin, but less pronounced that the enhancement of IL-17 and IL-1β.[6] This suggests that TNF-α, although present in inflammatory HS skin, may not be one of the big players in the pathogenesis of this disease. Overall, there is conflicting evidence in relation to the role of TNF-α in HS.

The data for IL-1β in HS, albeit from fewer studies, seem to be more consistent with IL-1β often one of the most enhanced cytokines demonstrated in various studies. IL-1β is a potent proinflammatory cytokine that drives the differentiation of Th17 cells.[18] Mature IL-1β is synthesized from its inactive precursor following cleavage by activated caspase-1, which in turn requires the assembly of a multiprotein complex known as the inflammasome. Activation of the inflammasome is implicated in several inflammatory disorders such as gout.[19] A 31-fold enhancement of IL-1β was demonstrated in HS lesional skin, and elevated concentrations were also observed in perilesional skin.[10] In another study by the same authors, a 54-fold increase in protein expression of IL-1β was observed.[17] A 115 fold enhancement of the mRNA expression of IL-1β in lesional and perilesional HS skin has recently been demonstrated and in this study it has been suggested that a subset of CD14+ dermal dendritic-cells produce IL-1β.[6] Wolk and colleagues[11] also documented enhanced mRNA expression of IL-1β, exceeding that of psoriatic skin. Meanwhile, the anti-inflammatory cytokine IL-10 has also been observed frequently in HS skin.[6,10,11,14,17] Its presence in involved skin is likely a response to a proinflammatory environment, although it is conceivable that high levels in lesional skin may have local immunosuppressive effects, therefore propagating inflammation and infection. Known cellular sources of IL-10 are activated T cells, macrophages, mast cells, and B lymphocytes that are abundantly present in HS lesional skin.[17]

The role of IL-17 in HS pathogenesis is emerging. IL-17 is produced by Th17 cells, which have a central role in many autoimmune diseases such as psoriasis and Crohn's disease.[20] Besides Th17 cells, innate lymphoid cells, γ-δ T cells, mast cells, and neutrophils have recently been shown to produce IL-17 also.[21,22] Th17 cell development is driven by IL-1β, IL-6, transforming growth factor-β, and IL-23, cytokines produced by activated innate cells such as dendritic cells.[20] Activated T cells, mast cells, and neutrophils are abundantly present in HS lesional skin. Schlapbach and colleagues[23] demonstrated IL-17 producing CD4+ T helper cells in HS lesional dermis, with protein expression of IL-17 enhanced by a factor of 30 compared with healthy controls. The same group also demonstrated that IL-23 was abundantly expressed by macrophages infiltrating the dermis in lesional HS skin. Wolk and colleagues[11] observed enhanced mRNA expression of IL-17 by a factor of 7, compared with control skin and similarly van der Zee and colleagues[17] documented a seven-fold enhancement in the protein expression of IL-17 analyzed following transwell culture. A recent study also demonstrated a 149-fold enhancement of mRNA expression of IL-17 in lesional skin. In addition, enhancement of IL-17 was documented in perilesional and clinically uninvolved skin (10 cm away from an active lesion) in HS patients, suggesting a primary role for immune dysregulation in HS.[6] CD4+ T cells were again documented as the cellular source of IL-17 in this study.[6] The detection of IL-1β, IL-23, and IL-17 therefore implicates the IL-1β-IL-23/Th17/IL-17 pathway in the pathogenesis of this disease.

IL-6 is a pleotropic key proinflammatory cytokine, but its role in HS pathogenesis remains undefined.[5] The IL-12/Th1 pathway was once considered pivotal in many inflammatory conditions until the discovery of Th17 cells. IL-12 has also been observed in a limited number of studies in HS skin. Remarkably however, interferon-γ, largely produced by Th1 cells, was not consistently seen in HS studies.[5]

ANTIMICROBIAL PEPTIDES

Constitutively produced antimicrobial peptides (AMPs), released as part of the body's innate immune response to microbial threat, are secreted by keratinocytes in large quantities in the presence of invasive pathogens.[24] In addition to antimicrobial properties, they also have immunomodulatory effects such as cytokine production, antigen presentation, recruitment of immune cells, and wound healing.[24] AMPs are particularly important where the skin barrier function is disrupted as a means of preventing or limiting cutaneous infection.

Several studies have evaluated AMPs in HS. All studies on AMPs in HS have limitations, because in all cases mRNA and protein expression were not measured in parallel in the same sample using robust techniques such as quantitative polymerase chain reaction (PCR) and enzyme-linked immunosorbent assay (ELISA). Wolk and colleagues[11] demonstrated a relative deficiency, at an mRNA level, of all measured AMPs (beta defensin [BD] -1, BD-2, BD-3, S100A7 [psoriasin], S100A8 [calgranulin A], and S100A9 [calgranulin B]) in HS lesions, and this attenuation was even broader than that seen in atopic dermatitis (AD), a condition long associated with suppressed AMP levels, hence the propensity for bacterial superinfection in AD. These authors relate this to a relative deficiency of IL-22 and IL-20 in HS. Schlapbach and colleagues[25] reported a relative deficiency of BD-2, thus facilitating colonization by bacteria. Enhanced mRNA expression of psoriasin was observed by this group, however. Hofmann and colleagues[24] also demonstrated suppressed BD-3 and RNase-7. Relative deficiencies of AMPs, namely BD-4 and BD-2, were also documented by other groups in lesional skin compared with healthy controls.[13,14] In contrast to this, however, Emelianov and colleagues[12] demonstrated enhancement of LL-37 (cathelicidin), psoriasin, and BD-3. Overall, the pattern of AMP aberrancy is unclear in HS, but there appear to be alterations in levels and functioning of AMPs. How they contribute to the initiation/propagation of HS remains to be elucidated.

PROPOSED INVOLVED SIGNALING PATHWAYS IN HIDRADENITIS SUPPURATIVA

Pathogen recognition receptors (PRRs) are germline-encoded, nonclonal binding sites for the recognition of microbes/infectious agents by the innate immune system. PRRs may be found in the cytoplasm or cell surface of immunocytes, or be secreted into the local and circulating fluids.[26] PRRs include toll-like receptors (TLRs), the nucleotide oligomerization domain (NOD) proteins, the RIG-like helicases, and the C type lectins.[27] The main functions of PRRs include proinflammatory signaling, complement activation, opsonization, phagocytosis, and regulation of apoptosis.[28] They recognize microbial motifs or pathogen-associated molecular patterns (PAMPs), including bacterial wall components, viral nucleic components, various proteins of flagellae, and fungal cell wall components.[27]

Several groups have investigated the role of TLRs in HS with varying results. Hunger and colleagues[29] reported enhanced expression of TLR2 at mRNA and protein levels, as well as C-type lectin in the epidermis and dermis. In contrast to this, Dréno and colleagues[14] suggested deficient innate immunity with suppressed expression of TLR2, TLR4, TLR3, TLR7, and TLR9 in HS skin compared to healthy controls. TLR expression in HS is therefore not fully defined. The role of bacteria in the initiation or propagation of HS is also unclear.[4] Despite the clinical appearance of infection, bacterial examination, commonly from superficial lesions, has frequently shown a mixed growth of commensal microbes.[30,31] This has been challenged, however, by a recent report whereby specific pathogens were isolated after broad and prolonged culturing. Specific antibiotic therapy resolved these cases of HS.[32] In line with this, a recent case report of long-standing refractory HS demonstrated an excellent clinical response to intensive intravenous linezolid and meropenem, yet disease flared quickly after withdrawal, implying that infection is not the primary etiology of this disease.[33] The suggestion is that there may be an overzealous TLR response to commensal bacteria as an initiating factor in the pathogenesis of HS, launching an inflammatory cascade.[4] Once HS is established, with sinus tract and fistula formation, secondary bacterial superinfection is likely to play a role in disease exacerbation, where bacterial colonies are harbored in these tracts in a biofilm formation, making eradication challenging and propagating inflammation.[34] Recent reports suggest that, at least in advanced stages of HS, superinfection with bacterial strains known to induce soft tissue infections may occur, which responds to intensive targeted antibiotic therapy.[32,33]

Advances in the genetics of HS have demonstrated loss of function mutations in 3 of the 4 subunits of γ-secretase, at least in a clinical subtype of familial HS.[35] γ-secretase cleaves the intracellular domain of Notch and Notch- signaling has many functions including the regulation of hair follicle differentiation and maintenance of the epidermal barrier.[35] Defective Notch signaling therefore occurs in HS, resulting in the inhibition of the hair growth cycle, the conversion of hair follicles into keratin-enriched epidermal cysts, and poor sebaceous gland differentiation.[36,37] Notch and TLR interaction has been reported, in which notch signaling suppresses TLR-4 induced proinflammatory cytokine responses by macrophages.[38] As this negative feedback is impaired with Notch deficiency a proinflammatory environment ensues. IL-22 deficiency, demonstrated previously in HS[11] may be linked to Notch deficiency, as IL-22 secretion by T cells is Notch dependent[36] (**Box 1**).

EFFECTS OF SMOKING ON KERATINOCYTES AND SKIN IMMUNITY: FACILITATING SKIN INFLAMMATION?

HS has been linked epidemiologically to cigarette smoking.[39] Tobacco smoke is composed of thousands of chemicals, some of which may have proinflammatory and oxidative properties.[40] These components (along with nicotine) activate keratinocytes (KCs) via at least 2 types of receptors: nicotinic acetylcholine receptors (nAChRs) and the aryl hydrocarbon receptors (AHRs).[41,42] Nicotine signals in an agonistic manner via the nAChR, expressed in the peripheral and central nervous system, as well as cutaneous keratinocytes, fibroblasts, and immunocytes.[41] In HS, nicotinic and tobacco smoke component stimulation of the KC cell cycle leads to acanthosis, infundibular epithelial hyperplasia, and excessive cornification.[43] The magnitude of activation depends on the expression of different nAChR subtypes. Nicotine can also alter host defense, thereby contributing to the pathogenesis of HS, including the generation of proinflammatory cytokines by keratinocytes, neutrophil chemotaxis, and Th17 cell induction.[4] Cigarette smoke generates a proinflammatory IL-1α/CXCR-2-dependent, aberrant neutrophilic response to bacteria in mice, where smoke-exposed mice were primed for excessive IL-1 production in response to bacterial ligands.[44] Moreover, nicotine favors the proliferation of *Staphylococcus aureus*, despite selective antimicrobial activity to other pathogens.[45] Coinciding with this, in HS the synthesis of antimicrobial peptides such as HBD-2 and S100A is suppressed in epithelial cells, rendering the host more susceptible to bacterial invasion.[11,25] Furthermore, tobacco smoke components enhance bacterial virulence by increasing cellular adhesion and inducing biofilm production.[46] Dioxins and polyaromatic hydrocarbons in cigarette smoke activate the AHR with resultant immunomodulatory effects including Th17 cell differentiation and expansion.[4] Down-regulation of Notch ligands, receptors, and downstream effector genes has recently been demonstrated in smokers, and this suggests that cigarette smoking, which is highly prevalent in HS, may further suppress already deficient Notch signaling in this disease[36] (**Box 2**).

Box 1
Defective Notch signaling sequelae

Defective Notch signaling: integrating genetics and biology

- Loss of function mutations in the γ-secretase gene are associated with HS
- γ-secretase cleaves intracellular Notch
- Defective Notch signaling is associated with the formation of follicular keratin-enriched epidermal cysts
- Notch negatively regulates TLR-4
- Defective Notch signaling will favor a pro-inflammatory environment

INFLAMMATORY PATHWAYS IN HIDRADENITIS SUPPURATIVA

A subclinical inflammatory state may arise in the skin prior to the onset of a visibly active HS lesion. It is suggested that the process begins with an aberrant keratinocyte response to commensal bacteria, which results in inappropriate cytokine and AMP production.[4] This results in a mild influx of immune cells, such as innate cells and T cells, which go on to secrete further proinflammatory cytokines and chemokines. The follicular epithelium

Box 2
Smoking and hidradenitis suppurativa pathogenesis

Contribution of smoking to HS pathogenesis

- Induction of epidermal hyperplasia
- Stimulation of follicular keratosis and occlusion
- Alteration of skin immune response (more neutrophilic)
- Increases microbial virulence
- Decreases skin antimicrobial peptides
- Down-regulation of Notch signaling

responds by becoming hyperplastic with keratosis of the infundibulum, follicular occlusion, and resultant cyst formation.[4] Smoking contributes to this process by promoting epidermal hyperplasia, and a proinflammatory environment.[4,41,44] Defective Notch signaling also produces keratin-enriched follicular cysts.[37] Cysts expand, rupture, and extrude contents into the dermis including corneocytes, bacteria, and keratin, triggering a neutrophilic foreign body reaction.[4] HS skin shows loss of periodic acid schiff-positive basement membrane in the pilosebaceous junction, so it is particularly vulnerable to rupture.[47] Histiocytic and multinucleated giant cells infiltrate and phagocytose free keratin. It is proposed that free keratin activates the NLRP3 inflammasome with caspase-1 mediated cleavage of pro-IL-1β into IL-1β, a potent proinflammatory cytokine.[4] Recently, caspase activation was demonstrated in HS lesional skin, with associated enhanced mRNA expression of NLRP3 in HS lesional skin compared to healthy control skin. Notably, active caspase-1 and NLRP3 activation is also required for synthesis of biologically active IL-18, and IL-18 was also demonstrated in both lesional and perilesional skin. Caspase-1 inhibition partly suppressed IL-1β and IL-18 secretion. Along with IL-23, IL-6, and TGF-β, IL-1β promotes the development of innate IL-17 and of Th17 cells, which in turn release IL-17, IL-22, and TNF-α.[20,48] An abundance of residual free keratin drives chronic responses with follicular epithelial strands remaining after cyst rupture to form fistulae-harboring bacteria and promoting suppuration[4] (**Fig. 1**).

SUMMARY

HS was once regarded a disease of primary infectious etiology.[41] This is understandable given the clinical presentation of recurrent painful nodules and abscesses, associated systemic malaise, elevated inflammatory markers, suppuration, exudation of serosanguineous material, and response to antimicrobials, at least in the short term. HS does not behave like a typical infection, however. Many cases do not ultimately respond to antibiotics, particularly more advanced, established chronic disease. HS is closely linked to other immune-mediated disease such as Crohn's disease and pyoderma gangrenosum, and responds to immunosuppressive agents such as oral corticosteroids and TNF-α inhibitors.[49] This suggests, at least in part, an immune basis for this disease, yet the exact mechanisms underpinning HS are not entirely established.[5]

It is now accepted that follicular occlusion is central to the pathogenesis of HS, and that apocrinitis is a secondary phenomenon.[1] Infundibular keratosis and follicular occlusion occur in the context of a genetic tendency, environmental factors, and immune aberrancy.[4] There is strong epidemiologic evidence that HS is highly associated with cigarette smoking and obesity.[39] The suggested mechanisms of smoking contributing to inflammation to HS have been outlined. Obesity is highly prevalent in the developed world, and most HS patients are overweight or obese.[39] Adiposity infers a low-grade proinflammatory state in which adipocytes secrete metabolically active proinflammatory cytokines known as adipokines,[50] which propagate the inflammatory cascade in this disease. Besides facilitating inflammation, adiposity also contributes to HS pathogenesis by increasing friction and follicular microtrauma at sites of predilection.[1] It has been suggested that a high systemic inflammatory burden may cause a state of insulin resistance, which is causally linked to endothelial dysfunction and atherosclerosis[51] and there is increasing evidence of an association with HS and the metabolic syndrome.[52]

The precise cytokine profile of HS has not been definitively elucidated; however, enhancement of IL-17, IL-1β, IL-10, TNF-α, and IL-23 has been demonstrated in various studies.[5] IL-1β, processed following activation of the inflammasome, is a potent inflammatory cytokine that has been demonstrated in high concentrations in HS.[5] An abundance of IL-1β may go on to promote the development of TH17 cells and subsequently IL-17 in HS.

Targeting IL-1β in HS is tempting yet reports of efficacy to date are conflicting. A case report and an open-label study suggest a benefit with anakinra, an IL-1 receptor antagonist.[53,54] Leslie and colleagues[54] documented a positive clinical

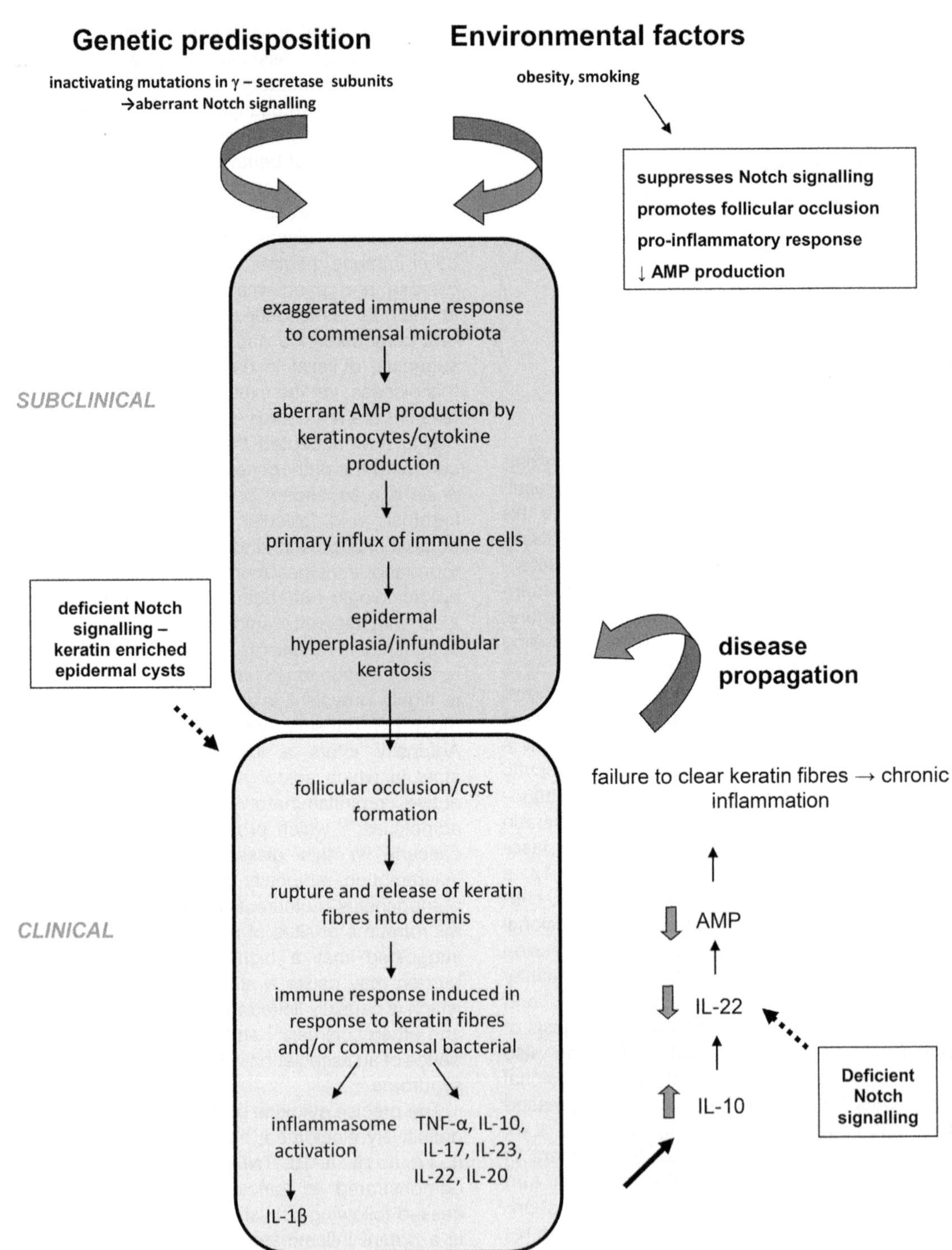

Fig. 1. Proposed pathogenesis in HS.

response in 5 of 6 patients treated with anakinra for 8 weeks, and this was reflected in functional T cell analysis. In contrast, however, there are a number of case reports of clinical failure with this drug.[55] Ustekinumab, an IL-12/23 inhibitor, may have a therapeutic benefit through ultimate blockade of Th1 and Th17 cell differentiation. Studies of ustekinumab in HS are limited, but Gulliver and colleagues[56] reported a benefit in 2 of 3 patients based on a visual analog scale of pain, physician global assessment, and dermatology life quality index. The effects of IL-17 blockade in

HS will be highly anticipated when these dugs become more widely available.

It is clear that HS is not simply a microbial disorder, as had once been thought. The role of bacteria in the initiation and/or propagation of HS is an area that warrants investigation, and new techniques should be employed to further assess the microbiome in HS. There are apparent parallels with other obesity-related processes (eg, diabetes, heart disease, cancer) where the interactions with the intestinal bacterial flora relate to proinflammatory activity.[57] This, along with the cytokine profiling outlined here, represent exciting fields of investigative endeavor likely to add to the therapeutic options available.

REFERENCES

1. Alikhan A, Lynch PJ, Eisen DB. Hidradenitis suppurativa: a comprehensive review. J Am Acad Dermatol 2009;60(4):539–61.
2. Scheinfeld N. Hidradenitis suppurativa: a practical review of possible medical treatments based on over 350 hidradenitis patients. Dermatol Online J 2013;19:1.
3. Revuz J. Hidradenitis suppurativa. J Eur Acad Dermatol Venereol 2009;23:985–98.
4. van der Zee HH, Laman JD, Boer J, et al. Hidradenitis suppurativa: viewpoint on clinical phenotyping, pathogenesis and novel treatments. Exp Dermatol 2012;21:735–9.
5. Kelly G, Sweeney CM, Tobin AM, et al. Hidradenitis suppurativa: the role of immune dysregulation. Int J Dermatol 2014;53:1186–96.
6. Kelly G, Hughes R, McGarry T, et al. Dysregulated cytokine expression in lesional and nonlesional skin in hidradenitis suppurativa. Br J Dermatol 2015. http://dx.doi.org/10.1111/bjd.14075. [Epub ahead of print].
7. O'Shea JJ, Ma A, Lipsky P. Cytokines and autoimmunity. Nat Rev Immunol 2002;2:37–45.
8. Grant A, Gonzalez T, Montgomery MO, et al. Infliximab therapy for patients with moderate to severe hidradenitis suppurativa: a randomized, double-blind, placebo-controlled crossover trial. J Am Acad Dermatol 2010;62:205–17.
9. Miller I, Lynggaard CD, Lophaven S, et al. A double-blind placebo-controlled randomized trial of adalimumab in the treatment of hidradenitis suppurativa. Br J Dermatol 2011;165:391–8.
10. van der Zee HH, de Ruiter L, van den Broecke DG, et al. Elevated levels of tumour necrosis factor (TNF)-α, interleukin (IL)-1β and IL-10 in hidradenitis suppurativa skin: a rationale for targeting TNF-α and IL-1β. Br J Dermatol 2011;164:1292–8.
11. Wolk K, Warszawska K, Hoeflich C, et al. Deficiency of IL-22 contributes to a chronic inflammatory disease: pathogenetic mechanisms in acne inversa. J Immunol 2011;186:1228–39.
12. Emelianov VU, Bechara FG, Gläser R, et al. Immunohistological pointers to a possible role for excessive cathelicidin (LL-37) expression by apocrine sweat glands in the pathogenesis of hidradenitis suppurativa/acne inversa. Br J Dermatol 2012;166:1023–34.
13. Mozeika E, Pilmane M, Nürnberg BM, et al. Tumour necrosis factor-alpha and matrix metalloproteinase-2 are expressed strongly in hidradenitis suppurativa. Acta Derm Venereol 2013;93:301–4.
14. Dréno B, Khammari A, Brocard A, et al. Hidradenitis suppurativa: the role of deficient cutaneous innate immunity. Arch Dermatol 2012;148:182–6.
15. Giamarellos-Bourboulis EJ, Antonopoulou A, Petropoulou C, et al. Altered innate and adaptive immune responses in patients with hidradenitis suppurativa. Br J Dermatol 2007;156:51–6.
16. Matusiak L, Bieniek A, Szepietowski JC. Increased serum tumour necrosis factor-alpha in hidradenitis suppurativa patients: is there a basis for treatment with anti-tumour necrosis factor-alpha agents? Acta Derm Venereol 2009;89:601–3.
17. van der Zee HH, Laman JD, de Ruiter L, et al. Adalimumab (antitumour necrosis factor-alpha) treatment of hidradenitis suppurativa ameliorates skin inflammation: an in situ and ex vivo study. Br J Dermatol 2012;166:298–305.
18. Sutton C, Brereton C, Keogh B, et al. A crucial role for interleukin (IL)-1 in the induction of IL-17-producing T cells that mediate autoimmune encephalomyelitis. J Exp Med 2006;203:1685–91.
19. Schroder K, Tschopp J. The inflammasomes. Cell 2010;140:821–32.
20. Maddur MS, Miossec P, Kaveri SV, et al. Th17 cells: biology, pathogenesis of autoimmune and inflammatory diseases, and therapeutic strategies. Am J Pathol 2012;181:8–18.
21. O'Brien RL, Born WK. Dermal $\gamma\delta$ T cells - What have we learned? Cell Immunol 2015;296(1):62–9.
22. Keijsers RR, Joosten I, van Erp PE, et al. Cellular sources of IL-17 in psoriasis: a paradigm shift? Exp Dermatol 2014;23:799–803.
23. Schlapbach C, Hänni T, Yawalkar N, et al. Expression of the IL-23/Th17 pathway in lesions of hidradenitis suppurativa. J Am Acad Dermatol 2011;65:790–8.
24. Hofmann SC, Saborowski V, Lange S, et al. Expression of innate defense antimicrobial peptides in hidradenitis suppurativa. J Am Acad Dermatol 2012; 66:966–74.
25. Schlapbach C, Yawalkar N, Hunger RE. Human beta-defensin-2 and psoriasin are overexpressed in lesions of acne inversa. J Am Acad Dermatol 2009;61:58–65.
26. Medzhitov R, Janeway CA Jr. Innate immunity: the virtues of a nonclonal system of recognition. Cell 1997;91:295–8.

27. Akira S, Uematsu S, Takeuchi O. Pathogen recognition and innate immunity. Cell 2006;124:783–801.
28. Janeway CA Jr, Medzhitov R. Innate immune recognition. Annu Rev Immunol 2002;20:197–216.
29. Hunger RE, Surovy AM, Hassan AS, et al. Toll-like receptor 2 is highly expressed in lesions of acne inversa and colocalizes with C-type lectin receptor. Br J Dermatol 2008;158:691–7.
30. Sartorius K, Killasli H, Oprica C, et al. Bacteriology of hidradenitis suppurativa exacerbations and deep tissue cultures obtained during carbon dioxide laser treatment. Br J Dermatol 2012;166:879–83.
31. Lapins J, Jarstrand C, Emtestam L. Coagulase-negative staphylococci are the most common bacteria found in cultures from the deep portions of hidradenitis suppurativa lesions, as obtained by carbon dioxide laser surgery. Br J Dermatol 1999; 140:90–5.
32. Guet-Revillet H, Coignard-Biehler H, Jais JP, et al. Bacterial pathogens associated with hidradenitis suppurativa, France. Emerg Infect Dis 2014;20: 1990–8.
33. Scheinfeld N. Extensive hidradenitis suppurativa (HS) Hurly stage III disease treated with intravenous (IV) linezolid and meropenem with rapid remission. Dermatol Online J 2015;21(2).
34. Kathju S, Lasko LA, Stoodley P. Considering hidradenitis suppurativa as a bacterial biofilm disease. FEMS Immunol Med Microbiol 2012;652:385–9.
35. Wang B, Yang W, Wen W, et al. Gamma-secretase gene mutations in familial acne inversa. Science 2010;330:1065.
36. Melnik BC, Plewig G. Impaired Notch signalling: the unifying mechanism explaining the pathogenesis of acne inversa. Br J Dermatol 2013;168:876–8.
37. Melnik BC, Plewig G. Impaired Notch-MKP-1 signalling in hidradenitis suppurativa: an approach to pathogenesis by evidence from translational biology. Exp Dermatol 2013;22:172–7.
38. Gentle ME, Rose A, Bugeon L, et al. Noncanonical Notch signaling modulates cytokine responses of dendritic cells to inflammatory stimuli. J Immunol 2012;189:1274–84.
39. Schrader AM, Deckers IE, van der Zee HH, et al. Hidradenitis suppurativa: a retrospective study of 846 Dutch patients to identify factors associated with disease severity. J Am Acad Dermatol 2014;71: 460–7.
40. Smith CJ, Hansch C. The relative toxicity of compounds in mainstream cigarette smoke condensate. Food Chem Toxicol 2000;38:637–46.
41. Kurzen H, Kurokawa I, Jemec GB, et al. What causes hidradenitis suppurativa? Exp Dermatol 2008;17(5):455–6 [discussion: 457–72].
42. Esser C, Rannug A, Stockinger B. The aryl hydrocarbon receptor in immunity. Trends Immunol 2009;30: 447–54.
43. Hana A, Booken D, Henrich C, et al. Functional significance of non-neuronal acetylcholine in skin epithelia. Life Sci 2007;80:2214–20.
44. Nikota JK, Shen P, Morissette MC, et al. Cigarette smoke primes the pulmonary environment to IL-1α/CXCR-2-dependent nontypeable Haemophilus influenzae-exacerbated neutrophilia in mice. J Immunol 2014;15(193):3134–45.
45. Pavia CS, Pierre A, Nowakowski J. Antimicrobial activity of nicotine against a spectrum of bacterial and fungal pathogens. J Med Microbiol 2000;49:675–6.
46. Hutcherson JA, Scott DA, Bagaitkar J. Scratching the surface - tobacco-induced bacterial biofilms. Tob Induc Dis 2015;13:1.
47. Danby FW, Jemec GB, Marsch WCh, et al. Preliminary findings suggest hidradenitis suppurativa may be due to defective follicular support. Br J Dermatol 2013;168:1034–9.
48. Sweeney CM, Tobin AM, Kirby B. Innate immunity in the pathogenesis of psoriasis. Arch Dermatol Res 2011;303:691–705.
49. Miller IM, Holzman RJ, Hamzavi I. Prevalence, risk factors, and co-morbidities of HS. Derm Clin, in press.
50. Nakamura K, Fuster JJ, Walsh K. Adipokines: a link between obesity and cardiovascular disease. J Cardiol 2014;63:250–9.
51. Boehncke WH, Boehncke S, Tobin AM, et al. The 'psoriatic march': a concept of how severe psoriasis may drive cardiovascular comorbidity. Exp Dermatol 2011;20:303–7.
52. Sabat R, Chanwangpong A, Schneider-Burrus S, et al. Increased prevalence of metabolic syndrome in patients with acne inversa. PLoS One 2012;7:e31810.
53. Zarchi K, Dufour DN, Jemec GB. Successful treatment of severe hidradenitis suppurativa with anakinra. JAMA Dermatol 2013;149:1192–4.
54. Leslie KS, Tripathi SV, Nguyen TV, et al. An open-label study of anakinra for the treatment of moderate to severe hidradenitis suppurativa. J Am Acad Dermatol 2014;70:243–51.
55. van der Zee HH, Prens EP. Failure of anti-interleukin-1 therapy in severe hidradenitis suppurativa: a case report. Dermatology 2013;226:97–100.
56. Gulliver WP, Jemec GB, Baker KA. Experience with ustekinumab for the treatment of moderate to severe hidradenitis suppurativa. J Eur Acad Dermatol Venereol 2012;26:911–4.
57. Patel S, Ahmed S. Emerging field of metabolomics: Big promise for cancer biomarker identification and drug discovery. J Pharm Biomed Anal 2015; 107C:63–74.

Imaging of Hidradenitis Suppurativa

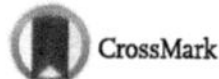

Ximena Wortsman, MD*

KEYWORDS

- Hidradenitis suppurativa • Hidradenitis suppurativa ultrasound • Hidradenitis imaging
- Hidradenitis MRI • Hidradenitis suppurativa color Doppler ultrasound
- Hidradenitis suppurativa sonography • Skin ultrasound • Dermatologic ultrasound
- Inflammation ultrasound • Hidradenitis staging

KEY POINTS

- Clinical examination alone can underestimate the severity of HS.
- Color Doppler ultrasound may support the management of hidradenitis suppurativa.
- Sonographic criteria for supporting the diagnosis are established.
- Disease staging is possible using ultrasound.
- MRI can help in the diagnosis of extensive and deep anogenital lesions.

Videos of Power Doppler and gray scale ultrasound accompany this article at http://www.derm.theclinics.com/

INTRODUCTION

Hidradenitis suppurativa (HS) is a complex disease of difficult management. The actual origin of the disease remains unclear. Moreover, according to a review by Rambhatla and colleagues[1] most therapies used to treat HS are only supported by limited or weak scientific evidence. Even though the diagnosis is mainly based on visual inspection, clinical assessment of the severity presents limitations. Thus, the usually used Hurley scoring relies only on clinical data, but lacks the accurate anatomic information necessary for use in clinical trials.[2] The Sartorius scoring seems to be time-consuming and relies on some clinical data that may be inaccurate and need modification after the use of imaging, such as the longest distance between two lesions separated by clinically normal skin.[3] Clinical interpretation of the nodules, abscesses, and fistulae may also be subject to reinterpretation under imaging. Palpation seems to be limited spatially because of the strong presence of inflammation and it may lead to misinterpretation of a fistula for a nodule, which can produce an erroneous assignment of the stage of severity and therefore the treatment.[4] Histology seems to be limited in HS because of the extensive and deep multiregional involvement.

The role of imaging in HS is to detect the actual type and extent of anatomic abnormalities by providing objective and precise information. Hence, it should support early diagnosis and assessment of severity of the disease. This may also include monitoring of treatment, presurgical mapping of lesions, and provision of detailed anatomic information for clinical trials. Furthermore, it has been demonstrated that the addition of imaging, particularly color Doppler ultrasound,

Disclosures: None.

Department of Radiology and Department of Dermatology, Institute for Diagnostic Imaging and Research of the Skin and Soft Tissues, Clinica Servet, Faculty of Medicine, University of Chile, Santiago, Chile
* Lo Fontecilla 201, of 734, Las Condes, Santiago, Chile.
E-mail address: xworts@yahoo.com

Dermatol Clin 34 (2016) 59–68
http://dx.doi.org/10.1016/j.det.2015.08.003
0733-8635/16/$ – see front matter

can significantly modify management in more than 80% of HS patients because of the clinical underestimation of severity.[4]

The first-line and most frequent imaging examination used for studying HS is color Doppler ultrasound. This imaging technique presents good resolution for studying the skin and deeper layers.[5] MRI has been mainly used in some extensive and deep anogenital HS lesions.[6] Nevertheless, MRI is expensive and currently the commercially available units present limitations in their resolution for detecting abnormalities in skin layers. However, it can observe the anatomic alterations in deeper structures.[7]

As with any medical test, the performance of imaging examinations requires adequate equipment and training of the operators that acquire the images and interpret the examinations. The latter is of paramount importance for standardizing the acquisition protocols and the categorization of lesions.[7,8]

Box 1
Ultrasound criteria for diagnosing hidradenitis suppurativa

1. Widening of the hair follicles
2. Thickening and/or abnormal echogenicity of the dermis
3. Dermal pseudocystic nodules (ie, round or oval-shaped hypoechoic or anechoic nodular structures)
4. Fluid collections (ie, anechoic or hypoechoic fluid deposits in the dermis and/or hypodermis connected to the base of widened hair follicles)
5. Fistulous tracts (ie, anechoic or hypoechoic bandlike structures across skin layers in the dermis and/or hypodermis connected to the base of widened hair follicles)

The presence of ≥3 findings is the sonographic criteria for diagnosing HS.

From Wortsman X, Moreno C, Soto R, et al. Ultrasound in-depth characterization and staging of hidradenitis suppurativa. Dermatol Surg 2013;39:1837; with permission.

ULTRASOUND

This is an imaging modality based on the propagation and return of sound waves in different tissues.[9] Ultrasound is a real-time and safe imaging method without reported adverse reactions. Usually, it does not require intravenous injection of contrast media and allows a rich and live interaction between the sonographer and patient.[7,8] The structures or tissues can be classified according to their echogenicity pattern into anechoic (ie, fluid-filled structures that allow the passage of the sound waves; black), hypoechoic (ie, dense fluid-filled structures or solid structures; gray), and hyperechoic (ie, solid structures that might present capillary vascularity, heavy calcium deposits, or exogenous materials; white). Each of the echogenicity categories presents variations according to a gray scale map and the structures are also identified according to some posterior artifacts that depend on the nature of the lesion or structure.[10] For example, fluid-filled lesions, such as cysts, present a posterior enhancement acoustic artifact (ie, increased transmission of the sound waves; a lighter area deep to the lesion). In contrast, strongly calcified lesions show a posterior acoustic shadowing artifact (ie, lack of transmission of the sound waves; a black shadow deep to the structure).[10] On color Doppler or power Doppler (ie, for slow flow detection) examination the blood flow patterns can be described in real time, which includes the type (arterial or venous) and the velocity of the flow (spectral curve analysis in centimeter per second).[7,8,11]

Ultrasound is a multiaxial imaging examination that can measure the structures in centimeters or millimeters along any axis. This can be useful in HS where, for example, the fistulous tracts tend to show a tortuous distribution that can follow several axes.

Nowadays, the most common types of ultrasound machines for studying HS are multichanneled equipment with high and variable frequency probes that vary in their upper frequency range between 15 and 22 MHz.[7,8] The main advantages of these machines are their good balance between

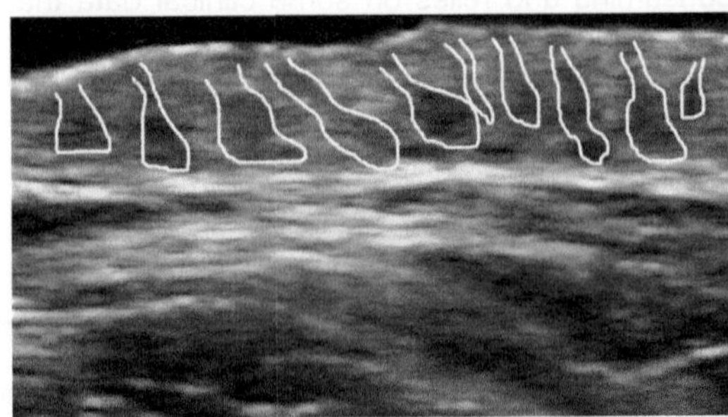

Fig. 1. Hidradenitis suppurativa widening of hair follicles. Ultrasound (gray scale, transverse view) shows widening of the bottom of the dermal hair follicles (*outlined*, "champagne bottle sign").

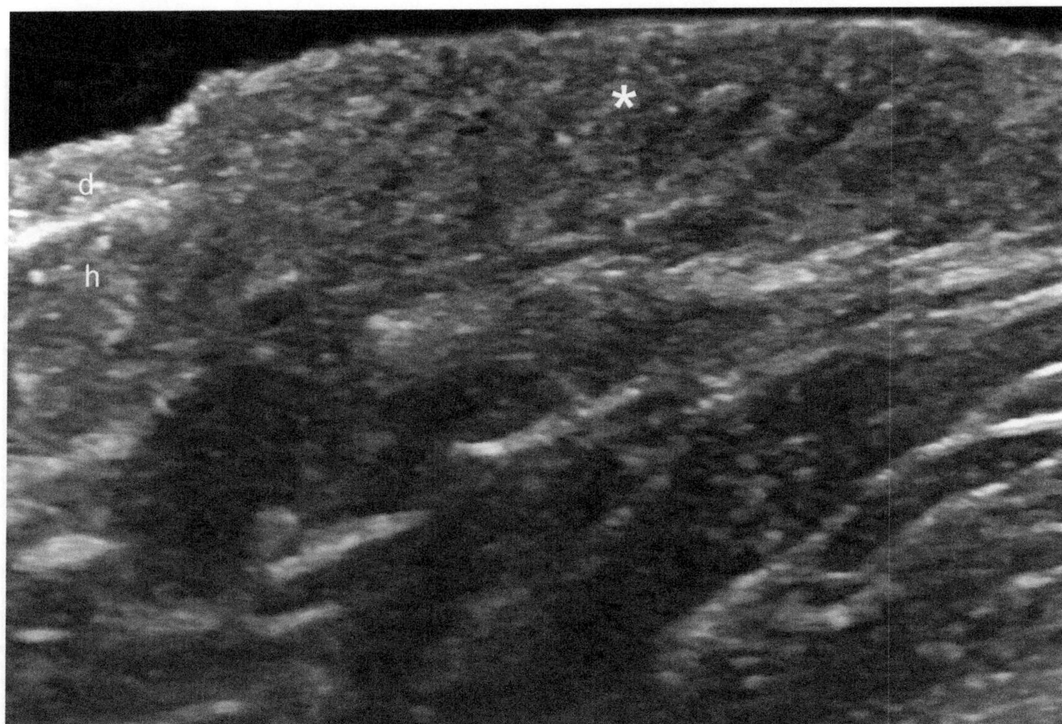

Fig. 2. Hidradenitis suppurativa dermal changes. Ultrasound (transverse view, left axillary region) shows thickening and hypoechogenicity of the dermis (*asterisk*) in comparison with normal skin (left aspect). d, dermis; h, hypodermis.

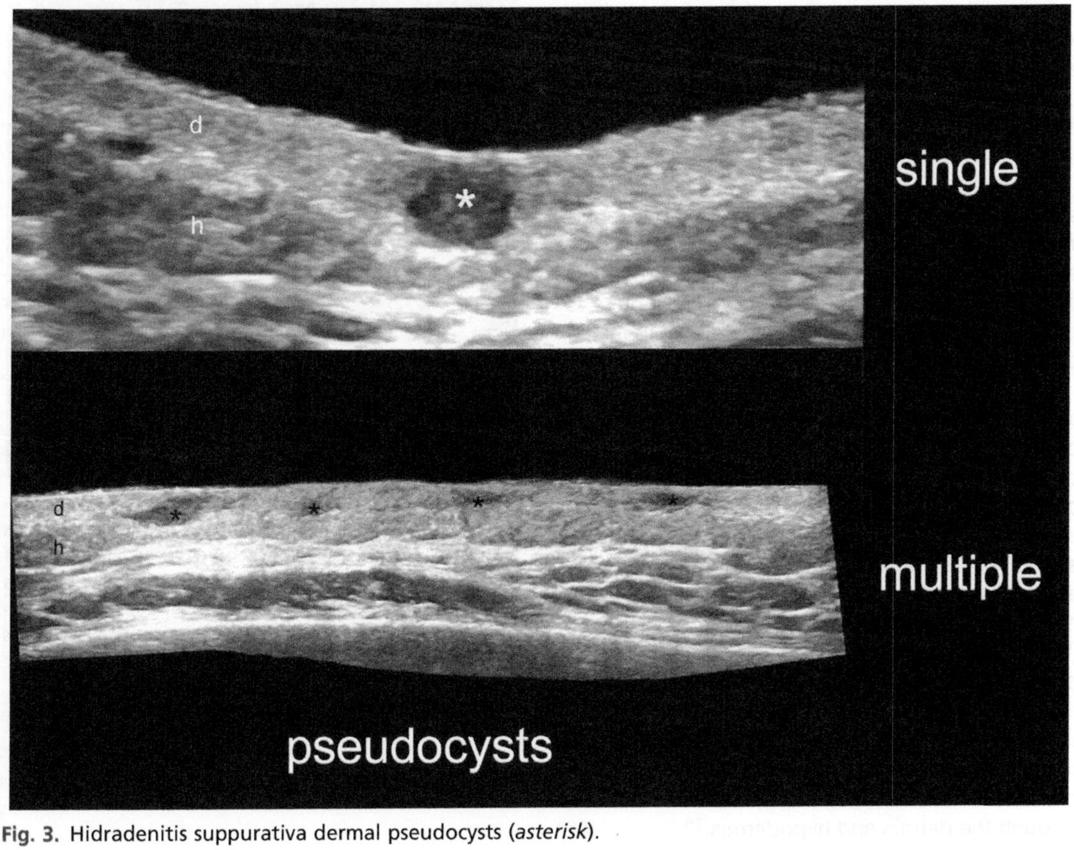

Fig. 3. Hidradenitis suppurativa dermal pseudocysts (*asterisk*).

resolution and penetration, which allows study of the skin and deeper layers without losing definition.[5,7,8] Additionally, their color Doppler capabilities allow clinicians to observe and follow the patterns of the lesional and perilesional vascularity, which can be signals for detecting and monitoring activity.[5,7,8] Currently, the limitations of this equipment are the detection of epidermal-only lesions, measuring less than 0.1 mm, and the detection of pigments.[5] Neither of these limitations seems particularly relevant for HS because of the usually dermal and hypodermal affection reported in this disease.[4]

On ultrasound, normal hair follicles appear as hypoechoic oblique dermal bands and the hair tracts present a predominantly trilaminar hyperechoic appearance in the scalp. However, in the rest of the body they tend to show a bilaminar or monolaminar hyperechoic linear pattern, which is compatible with the villus type of hair.[12,13]

The usage of ultrasound in HS started with 20-MHz compact ultrasound units that lack color Doppler during the 1990s. These allowed detection of the widening of the hair follicles in HS patients.[14] Later, with the development of high-frequency multichanneled color Doppler ultrasound machines the detection of subclinical abnormalities, such as echostructural dermal alterations (ie, increased thickness and decreased echogenicity), and the presence of anechoic or hypoechoic dermal and hypodermal fluid collections and fistulae were added to the detection of dilatation of the dermal hair follicles.[15]

Interestingly, on sonography it has been demonstrated that enlarged lymph nodes are rarely found in HS, and only appear involved in late and usually severe stages. It seems that this enlargement (ie, >1 cm transverse axis) of the lymph nodes is mainly secondary to an infection rather than the disease by itself.[16]

In 2010, Kelekis and colleagues[17] showed in a small series that ultrasound can be used for supporting the diagnosis and assessing the severity of the disease through registering two parameters: dermal thickness and echogenicity.

In 2012, the usage of three-dimensional ultrasound reconstructions in HS demonstrated early and more detailed morphologic alterations in the hair follicles, such as the widening of their bases ("champagne bottle sign"), the gathering of two or more hair follicles through their basal parts, the consistent communication of the fluid collections and fistula to the widened hair follicles, and the early development of fistulous tracts that depart from the base of the hair follicles and run through the dermis and hypodermis.[18]

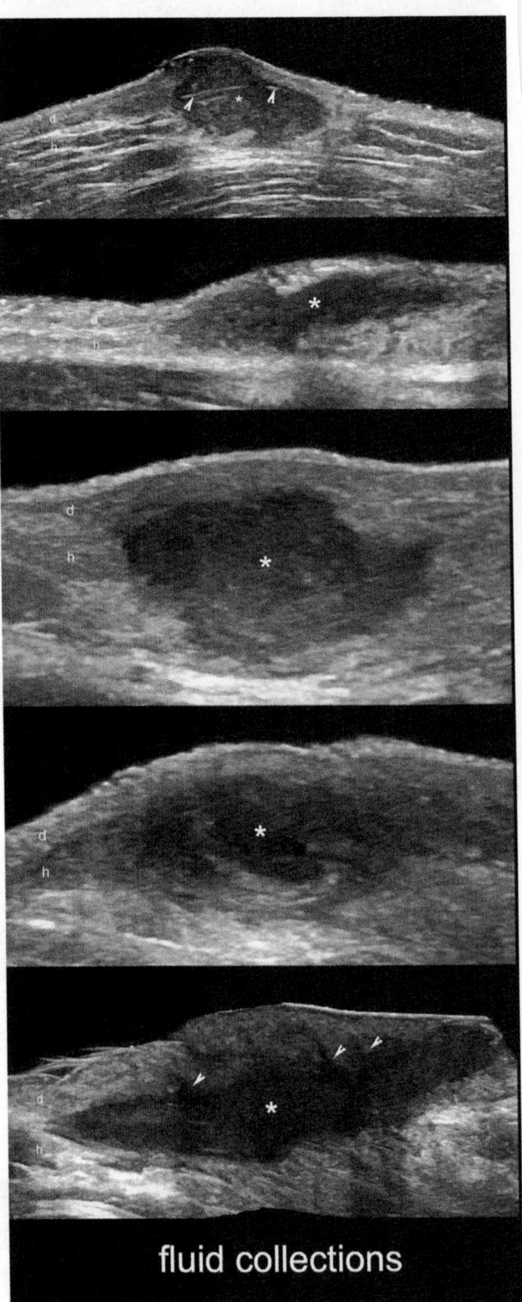

Fig. 4. Hidradenitis suppurativa variable presentations of dermal and hypodermal fluid collections (*asterisk*). Notice the hyperechoic linear fragments of hair tracts within the fluid collection (*top, arrowheads pointing up*) and the connections of the fluid collection to the bottom of widened dermal hair follicles (*bottom, arrowheads pointing down*).

In 2013, 16 years after the first report of ultrasound examination in HS,[14] the ultrasound criteria for diagnosing HS and a sonographic scoring system for assessing severity in HS (SOS-HS) were proposed.[4] This was mainly based on the presence of anatomic alterations, such as dermal echostructural abnormalities, and the recognition of dermal and/or hypodermal fluid collections and fistulae. Also, increased blood flow through low-velocity ($\leq$15 cm/s) arterial and/or venous vessels was frequently detected in the periphery of these fluid collections and fistulae.[4]

Another interesting sonographic finding is that patients' assessments of flare activity, pain, and erythema seem to be strongly associated with morphologic changes identified using ultrasound, suggesting that these items might be strong indicators of the degree of inflammation present in HS.[19]

As recently reported, the presence of retained fragments of hair tracts within the fluid collections and fistulae is an extremely common finding (Video 4; available online at http://www.derm.theclinics.com).[20] These variable size ectopic hair fragments seem to have lost their normal perpendicular vertical growth and outgrowth direction, and instead follow the axis of the skin layers. Probably, the presence of these nonreabsorbable keratin components that the human body does not recognize as foreign material allows the continuity and progression of the inflammatory process. Their actual role in the pathogenesis of the disease still remains to be determined; however, they seem to be linked to the persistent chronic evolution and the severity of HS.[20]

Ultrasound Criteria for Hidradenitis Suppurativa Diagnosis

The sonographic criteria for diagnosing HS are based on the following findings: widening of the hair follicles, dermal alterations, pseudocysts, fluid collections, and fistulae. The presence of three or more findings is the sonographic criteria for diagnosing HS (**Box 1**; **Figs. 1–8**) (Videos 1–3; available online at http://www.derm.theclinics.com).[4]

Using these criteria it has been reported that multiregional involvement occurs in two or more corporal segments in almost one-third (27%) of cases. Also there is a common presence of subclinical lesions that include fluid collections in 76%, fistulae in 29%, and dermal pseudocysts

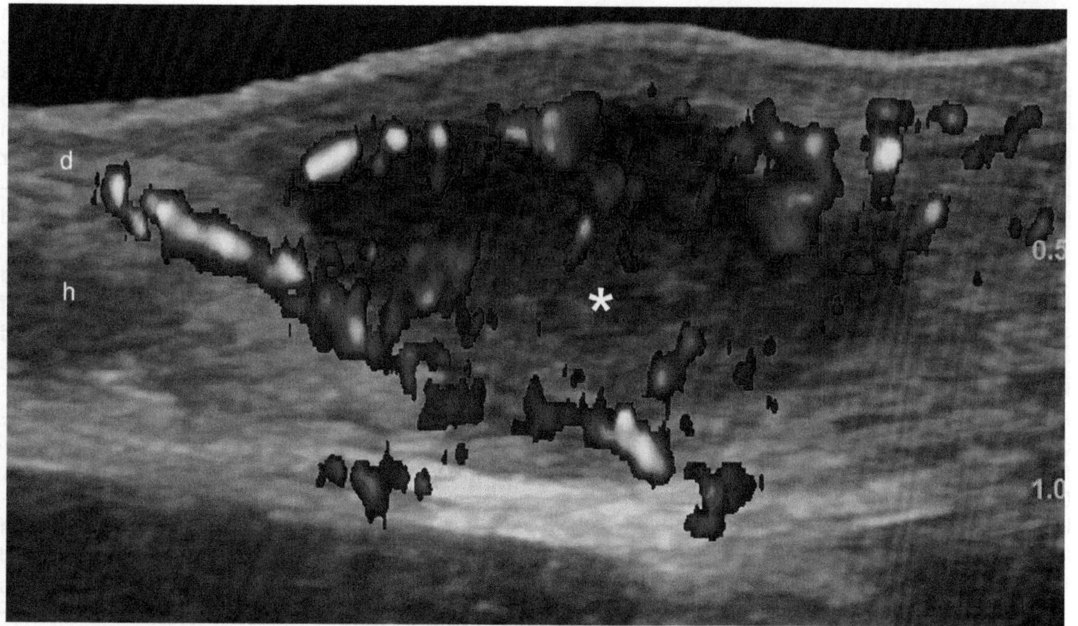

Fig. 5. Hidradenitis suppurativa active inflammation. Power Doppler (transverse view right groin region) demonstrates increased blood flow (*color*) in the periphery of a fluid collection (*asterisk*).

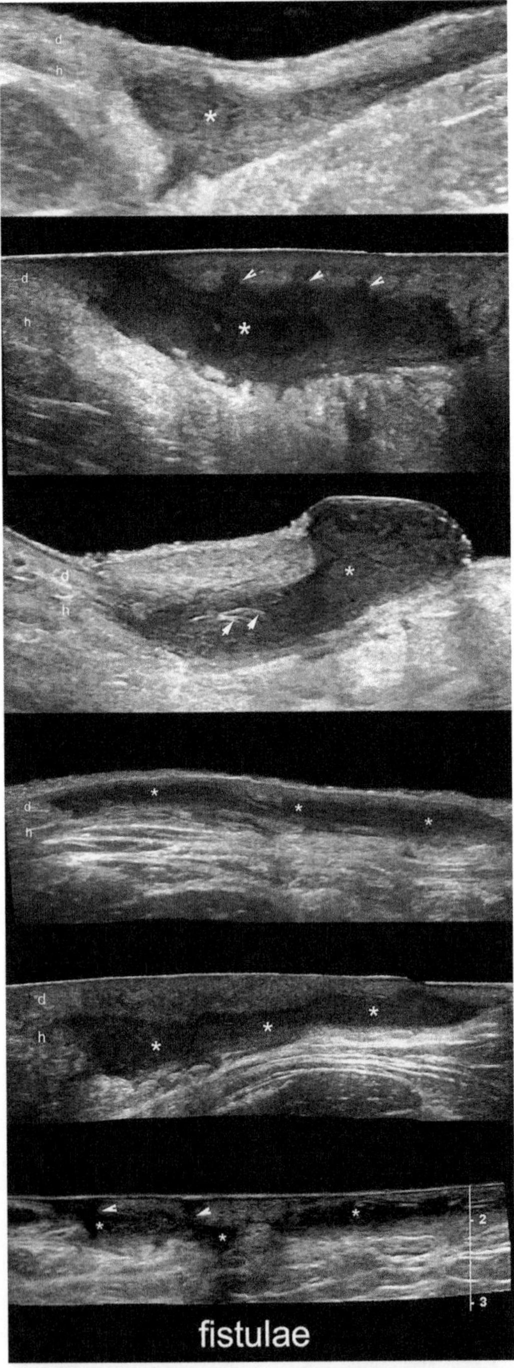

Fig. 6. Hidradenitis suppurativa variable appearances of fistulae (*asterisk*). Notice the connections of the fistulae to the bottom of widened hair follicles (*arrowheads pointing down*) and the hyperechoic linear fragments of hair tracts within a fistula (*arrows pointing up*).

in 71% of cases. Thirty-eight percent of patients show two to four collections ranging between 0.1 to 0.9 cm depth and 0.2 to 7 cm length. Twenty-nine percent of patients present fistulae that vary in their major axis between 1.7 to 12.2 cm and 0.02 to 1.1 cm in their thickness. The fluid collections and fistulae are usually located in the dermis and upper hypodermis and are connected to the base of widened hair follicles. According to the literature, the application of these ultrasound criteria has allowed a change in the clinical treatment in 82% of cases and the switch from medical to surgical management in 24% of cases.[4]

Ultrasound Staging

SOS-HS[4] (**Box 2**) mainly relies on the pivotal lesions that can potentially change the management of patients: fluid collections and fistulae. Thus, the performance of SOS-HS provides anatomic subclinical data that cannot be deduced from clinical examination. Besides dermal echostructural alterations and the number and distribution of fluid collections and fistulae, a description of their actual extent in all axes and vascularity (location, thickness, type, and velocity of the vessels) is usually performed. Therefore sonographic mapping and an index of activity of the lesions can be obtained.

The ultrasound technique for staging HS includes a sonographic sweeping of at least two different regions (eg, axillary and groin areas) in a sequential order that can go from top to bottom and from medial to lateral or lateral to medial according to the operator protocol. Once a lesion is detected it should be identified in at least two perpendicular axes and marked on the screen with a letter and a number (eg, C1 and C2 for collection and F1 and F2 for fistulae). These lesions are also measured in all axes and counted in each corporal region to achieve the final sonographic score.[4] The color Doppler ultrasound report usually includes a detailed description of the anatomic findings per regional segment and concludes with a summary and a sonographic score (SOS-HS).

MRI

This imaging modality relies on the exposure of tissues to a magnetic field. It provides a good definition of the hypodermis and deeper layers and allows examinations of the whole body.[21,22] Nevertheless, in the commercially available units the resolution for observing cutaneous layers is

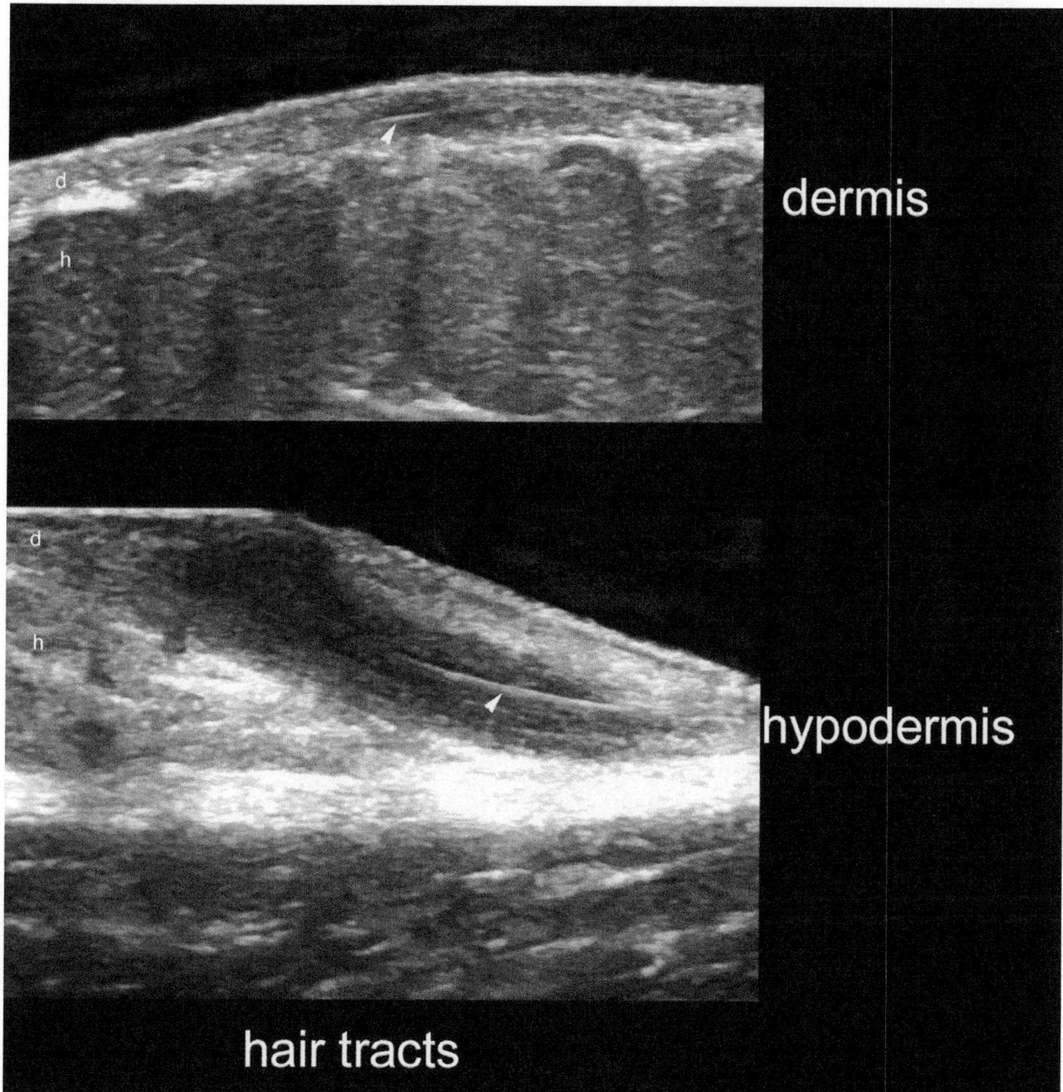

Fig. 7. Hidradenitis suppurativa retained hair tract fragments (ie, linear hyperechoic structures). (*Top*) In dermis. (*Bottom*) In the hypodermal part of a fistulous tract (*arrowhead*).

usually low and requires confinement of the patient to a reduced space during the examination. Also, intravenous contrast media is commonly injected, which may be the subject of potential adverse reactions. Among the secondary effects reported on MRI are nephrotoxicity and nephrogenic fibrotic dermopathy caused by the usage of gadolinium.[23,24]

Thus, MRI has been mainly used in the study of anogenital lesions in complex HS cases with prominent fistulous tracts or associated with other entities, such as Crohn disease.[6,25,26]

SUMMARY

Clinical examination alone can underestimate the severity of HS. Imaging, particularly color Doppler ultrasound, seems to be a powerful tool and the first imaging modality for supporting an early and more precise diagnosis and staging of severity in

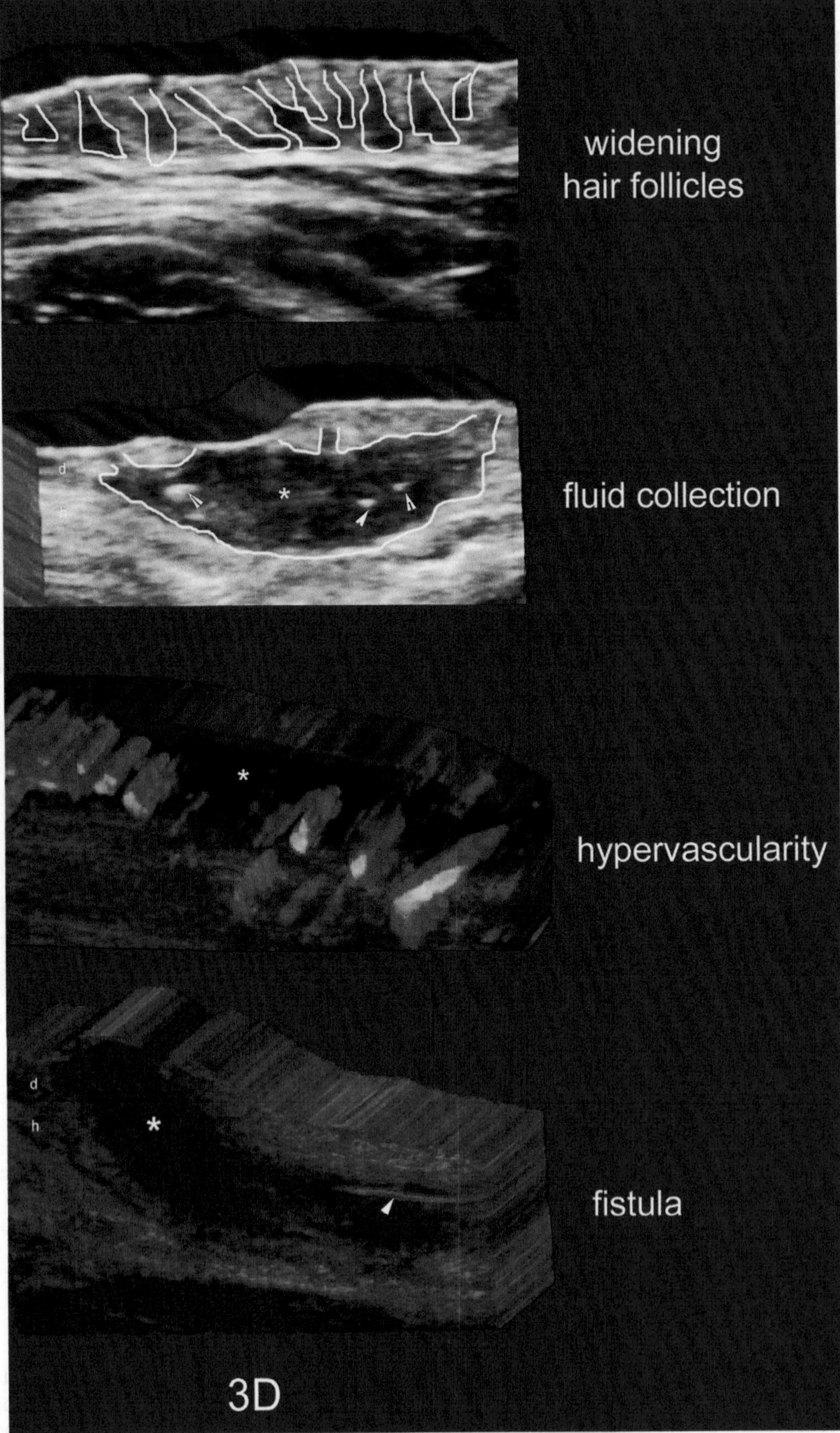

Fig. 8. Hidradenitis suppurativa three-dimensional ultrasound images showing the wide range of subclinical sonographic abnormalities. *, HS lesions; Arrowheads, fragments of hair tracts within the lesions.

Box 2
Sonographic Scoring of Hidradenitis Suppurativa

Stage I Single fluid collection and/or dermal changes[a] affecting a single body segment (either one side or bilateral), without fistulous tracts

Stage II Two to four fluid collections and/or a single fistulous tract with dermal changes, affecting up to two body segments (either one side or bilateral)

Stage III Five or more fluid collections and/or two or more fistulous tracts with dermal changes, and/or involvement of three or more body segments (either one side or bilateral)

[a] Dermal changes include hypoechoic or anechoic pseudocystic nodules, widening of the hair follicles, and/or alterations in the dermal thickness or echogenicity.

From Wortsman X, Moreno C, Soto R, et al. Ultrasound in-depth characterization and staging of hidradenitis suppurativa. Dermatol Surg 2013;39:1837; with permission.

HS. Additionally, because of the provision of detailed and objective anatomic data, imaging may help in the assessment of the pathogenesis of this complex disease and contribute to clinical trials.

SUPPLEMENTARY DATA

Supplementary data related to this article can be found online at http://dx.doi.org/10.1016/j.det.2015.08.003.

REFERENCES

1. Rambhatla PV, Lim HW, Hamzavi I. A systematic review of treatments for hidradenitis suppurativa. Arch Dermatol 2012;148:439–46.
2. Hurley HJ. Axillary hyperhidrosis, apocrine bromhidrosis, hidradenitis suppurativa and familial bening pemphigus: surgical approach. In: Roenigk RK, Roeningk HH, editors. Dermatologic surgery. New York: Marcel Dekker; 1989. p. 729–39.
3. Sartorius K, Killasli H, Heilborn J, et al. Interobserver variability of clinical scores in hidradenitis suppurativa is low. Br J Dermatol 2010;162:1261–8.
4. Wortsman X, Moreno C, Soto R, et al. Ultrasound in-depth characterization and staging of hidradenitis suppurativa. Dermatol Surg 2013;39:1835–42.
5. Wortsman X, Wortsman J. Clinical usefulness of variable frequency ultrasound in localized lesions of the skin. J Am Acad Dermatol 2010;62:247–56.
6. Griffin N, Williams AB, Anderson S, et al. Hidradenitis suppurativa: MRI features in anogenital disease. Dis Colon Rectum 2014;57:762–71.
7. Wortsman X. Common applications of dermatologic sonography. J Ultrasound Med 2012;31:97–111.
8. Wortsman X. Ultrasound in dermatology: why, how and when? Semin Ultrasound CT MR 2013;34:177–95.
9. Healy DA, Thiele BL, Neumyer MM. Current applications of duplex ultrasonography and color Doppler imaging. J Cardiovasc Surg (Torino) 1994;35:403–12.
10. Prabhu SJ, Kanal K, Bhargava P, et al. Ultrasound artifacts: classification, applied physics with illustrations, and imaging appearances. Ultrasound Q 2014;30:145–57.
11. Scoutt LM, Zawin ML, Taylor KJ, et al. Part II. Clinical applications. Radiology 1990;174:309–19.
12. Wortsman X, Wortsman J, Matsuoka L, et al. Sonography in pathologies of scalp and hair. Br J Radiol 2012;85:647–55.
13. Wortsman X, Guerrero R, Wortsman J. Hair morphology in androgenetic alopecia: sonographic and electron microscopic studies. J Ultrasound Med 2014;33:1265–72.
14. Jemec GB, Gniadecka M. Ultrasound examination of hair follicles in hidradenitis suppurativa. Arch Dermatol 1997;133:967–70.
15. Wortsman X, Jemec GBE. High frequency ultrasound for the assessment of hidradenitis suppurativa. Dermatol Surg 2007;33:1–3.
16. Wortsman X, Revuz J, Jemec GB. Lymph nodes in hidradenitis suppurativa. Dermatology 2009;219:22–4.
17. Kelekis NL, Efstathopoulos E, Balanika A, et al. Ultrasound aids in diagnosis and severity assessment of hidradenitis suppurativa. Br J Dermatol 2010;162:1400–2.
18. Wortsman X, Jemec G. A 3D ultrasound study of sinus tract formation in hidradenitis suppurativa. Dermatol Online J 2013;19:18564.
19. Zarchi K, Yazdanyar N, Yazdanyar S, et al. Pain and inflammation in hidradenitis suppurativa correspond to morphological changes identified by high-frequency ultrasound. J Eur Acad Dermatol Venereol 2015;29:527–32.
20. Wortsman X, Wortsman J. Ultrasound detection of retained hair tracts in hidradenitis suppurativa. Dermatol Surg 2015;41:867–9.
21. Deutsch AL, Mink JH. Magnetic resonance imaging of musculoskeletal injuries. Radiol Clin North Am 1989;27:983–1002.
22. Atkin KL, Ditchfield MR. The role of whole-body MRI in pediatric oncology. J Pediatr Hematol Oncol 2014;36:342–52.

23. Leander P, Allard M, Caille JM, et al. Early effect of gadopentetate and iodinated contrast media on rabbit kidneys. Invest Radiol 1992;27:922–6.
24. Moreno-Romero JA, Segura S, Mascaró JM Jr, et al. Nephrogenic systemic fibrosis: a case series suggesting gadolinium as a possible aetiological factor. Br J Dermatol 2007;157:783–7.
25. Kelly AM, Cronin P. MRI features of hidradenitis suppurativa and review of the literature. AJR Am J Roentgenol 2005;185:1201–4.
26. Koilakou S, Karapiperis D, Tzathas C. A case of hidradenitis suppurativa refractory to anti-TNFalpha therapy in a patient with Crohn's disease. Am J Gastroenterol 2010;105:231–2.

Randomized Controlled Trials for the Treatment of Hidradenitis Suppurativa

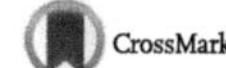

Dominique C. van Rappard, MD[a,*], Jan R. Mekkes, MD, PhD[a],
Thrasivoulos Tzellos, MD, MSc, PhD[b]

KEYWORDS

• Randomized controlled trials • Hidradenitis suppurativa • Treatment • Biologics • Surgery • Laser • Evidence based • Antibiotics

KEY POINTS

- Hidradenitis suppurativa (HS) is a chronic debilitating skin disease.
- High-quality evidence for the different treatment modalities of HS is lacking.
- Eleven randomized controlled trials are available concerning the treatment of HS.
- A variety of outcome parameters has been used, preventing indirect comparison.
- The need for appropriately designed randomized controlled trials is emphasized.

INTRODUCTION

Hidradenitis suppurativa (HS) is a chronic, inflammatory, recurrent, scarring, debilitating skin disease that usually presents after puberty.[1,2] HS also inflicts a significant burden on patients.[3,4] Epidemiologic studies also highlight that patients with HS present several cardiovascular risk factors, such as smoking, obesity, dyslipidemia (low high-density lipoprotein levels and hypertriglyceridemia), diabetes, and metabolic syndrome, at a significantly higher rate compared with healthy controls.[5–7] This evidence indicates that HS is more than a disease limited to skin and that it displays systemic chronic inflammation characteristics, like psoriasis.

In the evaluation of trials and reported treatment results, disease quantification is of the outmost importance. Hurley stage (**Table 1**), Modified Sartorius Score (MSS), and HS Physician's Global Assessment (HS-PGA) (**Table 2**) are measures that have been used to classify and assess HS disease severity (**Box 1**).[8–11] A new score was recently developed, evaluated, and validated as a clinical outcome for assessment of treatment effectiveness, especially for the inflammatory manifestations: the Hidradenitis Suppurativa Clinical Response (HiSCR).[12] The use of this validated, easy-to-use score is recommended in both research and daily clinical practice and it allows easier comparisons when assessing different trials. At present the inconsistencies in reported outcomes make such comparisons difficult.

A variety of treatment methods are available for HS, but only a few of them are based on high-quality evidence. This article gives an overview of

Disclosure: T. Tzellos has been reimbursed for travel expenses and hotel accommodation to attend dermatologic congresses by Janssen-Cilag, by MSD, and by Novartis. T. Tzellos also participates at the hidradenitis suppurativa advisory board of Abbvie. J.R. Mekkes has participated in clinical trials investigating infliximab and adalimumab in hidradenitis suppurativa, reimbursed by MSD and Abbvie.

[a] Department of Dermatology, Academic Medical Center, University of Amsterdam, Meibergdreef 9, Amsterdam 1105 AZ, The Netherlands; [b] Department of Dermatology, Faculty of Health Sciences, University Hospital of North Norway, Bjørnhågen 9, Harstad, 9407, Troms, Norway

* Corresponding author.

E-mail address: d.c.vanrappard@amc.uva.nl

Dermatol Clin 34 (2016) 69–80
http://dx.doi.org/10.1016/j.det.2015.08.012

Table 1
Hurley staging

Hurley Stage	Definition
I	Abscess formation, single or multiple, without sinus tracts and cicatrization
II	Single or multiple, widely separated, recurrent abscesses with tract formation and cicatrization
III	Diffuse or near-diffuse involvement, or multiple interconnected tracts and abscesses across the entire area

the currently available evidence for the pharmacologic as well as invasive treatment modalities of HS to facilitate rational decision making in daily clinical practice and elucidate recommendations for future randomized clinical trials.

METHODOLOGY

In order to objectively identify all randomized controlled clinical trials (RCTs) for the treatment of HS, a systematic search was undertaken in the electronic databases MEDLINE, EMBASE, and CENTRAL up to January 30 2015, using a draft search strategy for RCTs for MEDLINE (OVID), as suggested in the Cochrane Handbook.[13] Eligible criteria were RCTs that included patients with HS. Study designs other than RCTs were excluded. Conference abstracts and review articles were also excluded. There was a restriction for the English language. Information from each study was extracted using a standardized data extraction form. To assess the methodological quality, the Risk-of-bias tool suggested in the Cochrane Handbook for Systematic Reviews of Interventions was used.[13] The following items were critically appraised and extracted: method of generation of the randomization sequence, allocation concealment, blinding of participants, researchers and outcome assessors, incomplete outcome data (attrition bias), and selective reporting (reporting bias). In addition, the baseline characteristics

Box 1
How to evaluate patients with HS

Classification/severity assessment:

- Hurley stage
- MSS
- HS-PGA

Treatment effectiveness assessment:

- HiSCR (inflammatory manifestations)
- Inflammatory nodules, abscesses, and draining fistulas count

Comorbidities assessment:

- Quality of life (DLQI)
- Pain (VAS)
- Smoking
- Obesity (BMI, WC)
- Metabolic syndrome (NCEP-ATP III)
- Diabetes
- Anemia
- Dyslipidemia
- Work productivity (WPAI)

Abbreviations: BMI, body mass index; DLQI, Dermatology Life Quality Index; HiSCR, hidradenitis suppurativa clinical response; NCEP-ATP III, national cholesterol education program adult treatment panel III criteria; VAS, visual analog scale; WC, waist circumference; WPAI, work productivity and activity impairment questionnaire.

Table 2
HS-PGA

Clear (score = 0)	0 abscesses, 0 draining fistulas, 0 inflammatory nodules, and 0 noninflammatory nodules
Minimal (score = 1)	0 abscesses, 0 draining fistulas, 0 inflammatory nodules, and presence of noninflammatory nodules
Mild (score = 2)	0 abscesses, 0 draining fistulas, and 1–4 inflammatory nodules; or 1 abscess or draining fistula and 0 inflammatory nodules
Moderate (score = 3)	0 abscesses, 0 draining fistulas, and ≥5 inflammatory nodules; or 1 abscess or draining fistula and ≥1 inflammatory nodule; or 2–5 abscesses or draining fistulas and <10 inflammatory nodules
Severe (score = 4)	2–5 abscesses or draining fistulas and ≥10 inflammatory nodules
Very severe (score = 5)	>5 abscesses or draining fistulas

of study groups were checked for confounding factors in order to rule out selection bias.

RESULTS

The systematic search provided 197 results. After screening, 11 studies met the inclusion criteria. The selection process is summarized in **Fig. 1**. General study characteristics are summarized in **Table 3** and the most important results in **Table 4**. Four studies involved biologic therapy with anti–tumor necrosis factor (TNF) alpha. Two studies investigated the role of antibiotics, and 1 study investigated hormonal therapy. Also, 3 studies on laser treatment and 1 study of surgical treatment were included. The methodological quality of all studies is separately presented in **Fig. 2** and pooled in a graph in **Fig. 3**.

Biologics

The first RCT on biologics for HS involved infliximab, followed by 1 study on etanercept.[19,20] Subsequently 2 studies investigated the efficacy of adalimumab.[11,22] The positive effect of infliximab treatment was found by Grant and colleagues,[20] who studied 38 patients in a well-conducted, double-blinded trial lasting 52 weeks. Patients received infliximab (5 mg/kg at weeks 0, 2, and 6, and subsequently every 8 weeks) or placebo. After 8 weeks the double-blind phase was followed by an open-label phase in which patients taking placebo were given the opportunity to cross over. More patients in the infliximab group showed a 50% or greater decrease from baseline in HS severity score (a nonvalidated composite scoring system) compared with placebo at week 8, although this difference in improvement was not significant (27% vs 5%; P = .092). However, infliximab was significantly more effective on Physician's Global Assessment (PGA), visual analog scale (VAS), Dermatology Life Quality Index (DLQI), and in producing 25% to 50% improvement on HS severity score. Also, a significant reduction in inflammatory markers was observed at week 8. Infliximab monotherapy was well tolerated, and a greater number of adverse events occurred in the placebo group. Adverse events in the infliximab group were mild and included influenzalike illness, myalgia, dizziness, and headache. Also, 2 serious adverse events were reported, including pregnancy and hypertension. Adverse events in the placebo group included nausea, influenzalike illness, pyrexia, nasopharyngitis, and dizziness. One serious adverse event occurred, namely an infusion reaction.

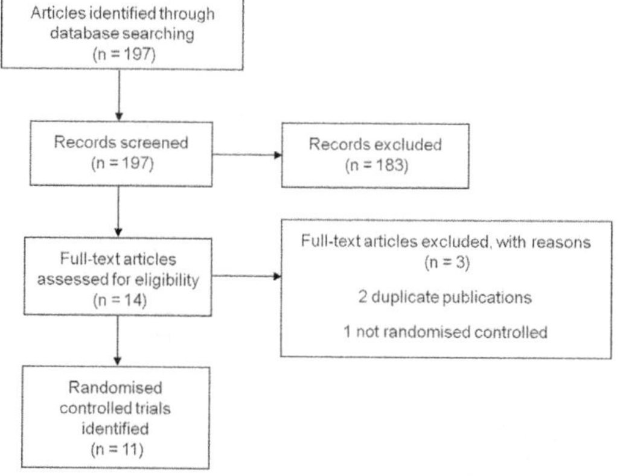

Fig. 1. Search strategy. Eleven RCTs were identified and included in this review. The general characteristics of these studies are included in **Table 3**.

Etanercept turned out not to be effective in a small RCT. Adams and colleagues[19] investigated 20 patients assigned to either etanercept 50 mg subcutaneously twice a week, or placebo for 12 weeks. Subsequently, all patients received open-label etanercept for 12 more weeks. There was no statistically significant difference in PGA between treatment and placebo groups (P>.99). Also, none of the secondary outcomes, including PGA and DLQI, were significantly improved. The only adverse drug reactions reported were mild injection site reactions, but it was unclear whether this occurred in both groups. A limitation of the study is the small, unjustified sample size and the brief description of trial design and outcome.

For adalimumab, Miller and colleagues[22] initially studied 21 patients with moderate to severe HS in a double-blinded, placebo-controlled trial. Actively treated patients received adalimumab 80 mg subcutaneously at baseline followed by 40 mg subcutaneously every other week for 12 weeks. A significant reduction was seen in Sartorius score after 6 weeks but not after 12 weeks (−10.7 vs 7.5, P = .02; and −11.3 vs 5.8, P = .07) compared with the placebo group. None of the secondary end points, including VAS pain and DLQI scores, reached statistical significance. More adverse events were observed in the adalimumab group, but this was not significantly different from placebo. The study observed an overall pattern of disease evolution and the investigators speculated that the dosage used may have been suboptimal. A limitation of this study was that it was underpowered because of early termination of recruitment because of expiration of trial medication, and because there was a difference in disease severity at baseline.

Subsequently, the optimal dosage was investigated by Kimball and colleagues[11] in a 3-arm, well-conducted RCT in 154 patients. The study

Table 3
Characteristics of RCTs for the treatment of HS

Citation	Setting	Methods	Patients	Intervention Groups	Control Group	Limitations
Clemmensen,[14] 1983	Denmark	Single-center, double-blind, placebo-controlled trial	30 patients with HS Hurley I and mild Hurley II	13 Topical CL 1% (dosing schedule unknown) for 12 wk	14 PL for 12 wk	Unjustifiable sample size, no intention-to-treat analysis
Mortimer et al,[15] 1986	United Kingdom	Single-center, double-blind, controlled, crossover trial	24 F patients with HS with moderate to severe HS	10 oral ethinyl estradiol 50 μg/CPA 50 mg (each menstrual cycle) for 12 mo (with crossover at 6 mo)	8 oral ethinyl estradiol 50 μg/norgestrel 500 μg (each menstrual cycle) for 12 mo (with crossover at 6 mo)	Unjustifiable sample size, no intention-to-treat analysis
Jemec & Wendelboe,[16] 1998	Denmark	Single-center, randomized, double-blind, controlled trial	46 patients with HS (39 F, 7 M), Hurley I and II	16 (13 F, 3 M) oral TCN 500 mg bid plus topical PL, minimum of 3 mo	18 (15 F, 3 M) topical CL 1% bid plus oral PL, minimum of 3 mo	Unjustifiable sample size, no intention-to-treat analysis
Buimer et al,[17] 2008	Netherlands	Single-center, randomized, controlled trial	200 patients with HS	124 (108 F, 16 M) surgical excision with PC plus GC	76 (72 F, 4 M) surgical excision with PC alone	No clear assessment of baseline severity
Mahmoud et al,[18] 2010	United States	Single-center, randomized, controlled split-body trial	22 patients with HS (19 F, 3 M), Hurley II	Nd:YAG laser monthly for 4 mo plus BP wash 10% and CL 1% lotion	BP wash 10% and CL 1% lotion alone	No clear report on side effects
Adams et al,[19] 2010	United States	Single-center, randomized, double-blind, placebo-controlled trial	20 patients with HS with moderate to severe HS	10 (6 F, 4 M), ETA SC 50 mg twice/wk for 12 wk	10 (7 F, 3 M), PL SC 50 mg twice/wk for 12 wk	Unjustifiable sample size

Grant et al,[20] 2010	United States	Single-center, randomized, double-blind, placebo-controlled, crossover trial	38 patients with HS with moderate to severe HS	15 (12 F, 3 M) IFX (5 mg/kg) IV on wk 0, 2, and 6	23 (14 F, 9 M) PL (5 mg/kg) IV on wk 0, 2, and 6 (with crossover at 8 wk)	—
Highton et al,[21] 2011	United Kingdom	Single-center, randomized, controlled split-body trial	18 HS (15 F, 3 M) patients, Hurley II and III	IPL twice/wk for 4 wk	No treatment	Unjustifiable sample size, no clear report on side effects
Miller et al,[22] 2011	Denmark	Two-center, randomized, double-blind, placebo-controlled trial	21 patients with HS with moderate to severe HS	15 (12 F, 3 M) ADA SC 80 mg at baseline, 40 mg eow for 12 wk	6 (5 F, 1 M) PL SC 80 mg at baseline, 40 mg eow for 12 wk	Early termination of recruitment, difference in baseline severity
Kimball et al,[11] 2012	United States, Denmark, Netherlands, Germany	Multicenter, randomized, double-blind, placebo-controlled trial	154 patients with HS with moderate to severe HS	51 (36 F, 15 M) ADA SC 160 mg wk 0, 80 mg wk 2, 40 mg weekly for 16 wk 52 (38 F, 14 M) ADA SC 80 mg wk 0, 40 mg eow for 16 wk	51 (36 F, 15 M) PL for 16 wk	—
Fadel & Tawfik,[23] 2015	Egypt	Single-center, randomized, controlled, split-body trial	10 patients with HS (7 F, 3 M) 4 Hurley I, 4 Hurley II, 2 Hurley III	NMB gel plus IPL, twice monthly, maximum 6 mo	Free NMB gel plus IPL, twice monthly, maximum of 6 mo	Unjustifiable sample size

Abbreviations: ADA, adalimumab; bid, twice daily; BP, benzoyl peroxide; CL, clindamycin; CPA, cyproterone acetate; eow, every other week; ETA, etanercept; F, female; GC, gentamicin-collagen sponge; IFX, infliximab; IPL, intense pulsed light; IV, intravenous; M, male; Nd:YAG, long-pulsed neodymium:yttrium-aluminum-garnet; NMB, niosomal methylene blue; PC, primary closure; PL, placebo; SC, subcutaneous; TCN, tetracycline.

Table 4
Results of RCTs for the treatment of HS

Citation	Primary Outcome (Time of Main Assessment)	Results	*P*-Value	Secondary Outcomes	Safety Assessment
Clemmensen,[14] 1983	Cumulative score of patients' assessment, number of abscesses, inflammatory nodules, and pustules (monthly)	Clindamycin more effective after every monthly assessment (+311 vs −91 after 3 mo)	<.01	None	No side effects, except for local slight burning pain after application (2 CL, 3 PL)
Mortimer et al,[15] 1986	Cumulative score based on patients' and observers' assessments (12 mo)	No difference	NR	PaGA on VAS, laboratory androgen assessment	CPA: 5 patients with symptoms of weight gain, headaches, and breast soreness Norgestrel: 8 patients with nonspecific side effects
Jemec & Wendelboe,[16] 1998	PaGA on VAS (monthly)	No difference	NR	PGA on VAS, soreness on VAS, counting of abscesses, counting of nodules	Oral TCN: 2 patients with gastrointestinal upset Topical CL: 1 patient with suspected allergic reaction
Buimer et al,[17] 2008	Percentage of postoperative complications, including dehiscence, infection, and seroma (1 wk)	Fewer complications for PC plus GC (35% vs 52%)	<.03	Local recurrence rate, wound healing duration, percentage recovery in 2 mo (assessed after 3 mo)	NR
Mahmoud et al,[18] 2010	Modified HS-LASI, based on Sartorius Score, percentage change from baseline (6 mo)	More improvement on site treated with Nd:YAG (−72.7% vs −22.9%)	<.001	Posttreatment questionnaire for patients, including pain, satisfaction, disease activity, and effectiveness Histopathologic examination	NR

Adams et al,[19] 2010	PGA of clear or mild (12 wk)	No difference	>.99	PaGA, DLQI, patients' pain scale	Only mild injection site reactions, not specified for which group
Grant et al,[20] 2010	HSSI>50% decrease from baseline, based on number of sites, body surface, number of lesions, drainage, pain VAS (8 wk)	No difference	.092	PGA, DLQI, VAS, laboratory markers (ESR and CRP)	More AEs in the PL group vs IFX, more serious AEs in the IFX group (pregnancy, hypertension) vs PL (infusion reaction)
Highton et al,[21] 2011	Sartorius Score, percentage change from baseline (12 mo)	More improvement on the site treated with IPL (−33% vs +3%)	<.001	Patients' satisfaction on a Likert scale	No complications
Miller et al,[22] 2011	Sartorius Score, change from baseline (12 wk)	No difference (−11.3 vs 5.8)	.07	Hurley Score, VAS, DLQI, self-reported days with lesions, scar scoring by patient and physician	More AEs in the ADA group vs PL group with regard to mild infections (P = .06)
Kimball et al,[11] 2012	HS-PGA, percentage patients achieving clear, minimal, or mild (16 wk)	Higher for ADA weekly (17.6% vs 3.9%), no difference for ADA eow (9.6% vs 3.9%)	.025 (weekly) .25 (eow)	MSS, Hurley Score, VAS, DLQI, WPAI-SHP, PHQ-9, CRP	15 serious AEs during exposure to adalimumab
Fadel & Tawfik,[23] 2015	Modified HS-LASI, based on Sartorius Score, percentage reduction in lesion size (time of assessment unclear)	NMB gel produced a higher percentage reduction in lesion size (77.3% vs 44.1%)	<.01	None	No side effects

Abbreviations: AE, adverse event; CRP, C-reactive protein; DLQI, Dermatology Life Quality Index; eow, every other week; ESR, erythrocyte sedimentation rate; HS-LASI, Hidradenitis Suppurativa Lesion Area and Severity Index; HSSI, Hidradenitis Suppurativa Severity Index; NMB, niosomal MB; NR, not reported; PaGA, patients' global assessment; PC, primary closure; PGA, physician global assessment; PHQ-9, Patient Health Questionnaire-9; PL, placebo; VAS, visual analog scale; WPAI-SHP, Work Productivity and Activity Impairment–specific Health Problem Questionnaire.

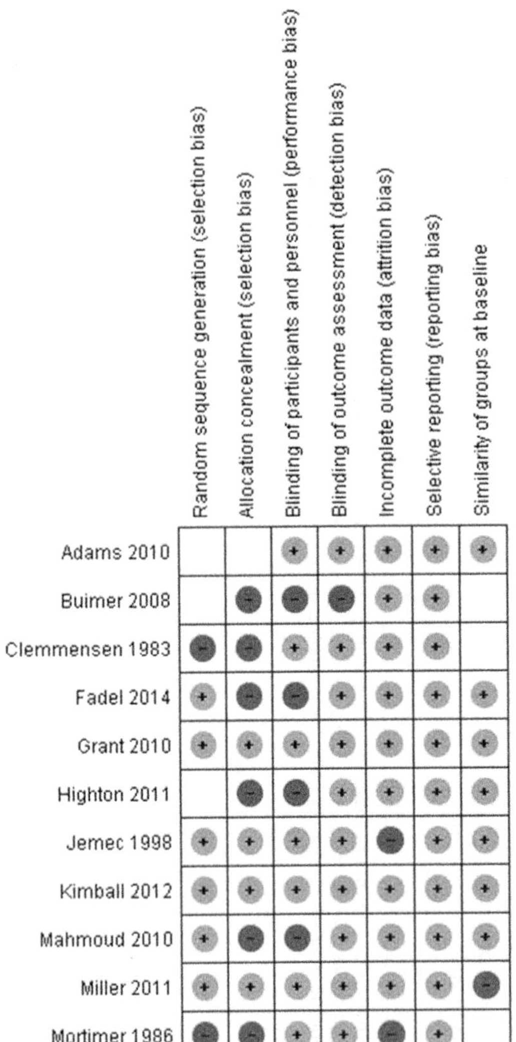

Fig. 2. Risk of bias: authors' judgments about each risk-of-bias item for each study.

consisted of a double-blind phase and an open-label phase. Patients were assigned to adalimumab 40 mg every week (after 160 mg at week 0, and 80 mg at week 2), 40 mg every other week (after 80 mg at week 0), or placebo. At week 16, the proportions of patients achieving a PGA score of clear, minimal, or mild, with at least a 2-grade improvement relative to baseline, were 17.6%, 9.6%, and 3.9% for every week, every other week, and placebo, respectively. A significant difference was only seen in the every-week group compared with placebo (*P* = .025), but not for patients randomly assigned to every other week (*P* = .25). Significant improvements were also seen in secondary outcomes, including VAS pain and DLQI, for the every-week group. A decrease in response was seen after the switch from every week to every other week in the open-label period. Kimball and colleagues[24] also presented a thorough and structured safety analysis. For the phase 2 trial of adalimumab, the number needed to treat (NNT) for the newly introduced outcome of HiSCR at week 16 was 4 (95% confidence interval [CI], 2.1–10.7), whereas the number needed to harm (NNH) for any serious adverse event was 26. This NNT to NNH ratio is favorable. This study concluded that adalimumab dosed every week alleviates moderate to severe HS, and therefore confirms the hypothesis of Miller and colleagues[22] that a higher dosage is needed to obtain an optimal treatment efficacy.

Antibiotics

Two RCTs were found concerning the use of antibiotics for HS, and both included topical clindamycin.[14,16] Clemmensen[14] investigated the use of topical clindamycin 1% solution versus placebo

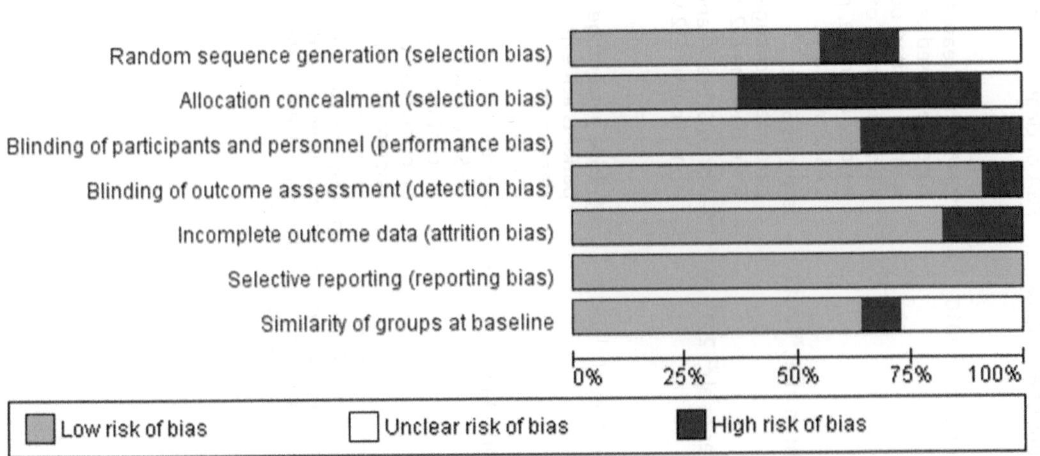

Fig. 3. Risk of bias: authors' judgments about each risk-of-bias item presented as percentages across all included studies.

in a double-blind, placebo-controlled trial in 30 patients. A significant difference in a nonvalidated, cumulative score, based on patient assessment, number of abscesses, inflammatory nodules, and pustules, was found after each monthly evaluation. A positive difference in score indicated improvement. After 3 months the difference in cumulative score was +311 for the clindamycin group and −91 for the placebo group (*P*<.01). When each parameter was evaluated separately, clindamycin was not superior for inflammatory nodules and abscesses. This finding was probably caused by the initial sparse number of lesions. No side effects were observed, except for a local slight burning pain after application in 5 cases, of which 3 patients received placebo. Limitations of the study included an unjustifiable sample size and that there was no intention-to-treat analysis.

Jemec and Wendelboe[16] compared topical clindamycin 1% solution twice daily with oral tetracycline 500 mg twice daily in 46 patients for a minimum of 3 months in a double-blind, double-dummy trial. Patients in both groups showed improvement from baseline, but no significant difference in efficacy between the two treatments was found. Patients' global assessment was significantly worse than physician's assessment, and soreness was the key factor in patients' overall assessment of disease. Therefore, the investigators concluded that soreness and other subjective factors should be included as outcome variables in future therapy studies. An increased consensus between patients' and physicians' assessments was observed later in the study. No information was provided on side effects, except for 2 patients who discontinued the study because of gastrointestinal upset and 1 patient with a suspected allergic reaction to topical clindamycin. In general, there was a high dropout rate, with twice as many dropouts in the systemic treatment group. Comparable with the study of Clemmensen,[14] no justification of the sample size was provided and no intention-to-treat analysis was performed.

Hormones

Mortimer and colleagues[15] allocated 24 patients in 2 groups matched for age and disease duration, and compared oral ethinyl estradiol 50 μg/cyproterone acetate 50 mg with ethinyl estradiol 50 μg/norgestrel 500 μg. The treatment was given sequentially for 12 months with crossover at 6 months. Both treatment arms improved compared with baseline, and there was no significant difference between the two groups. There was a high dropout rate. Side effects were mostly nonspecific in the case of norgestrel, but cyproterone acetate seemed to cause weight gain, headaches, and breast soreness. Based on the results that 7 patients cleared, 5 improved, 4 remained unchanged, and 2 deteriorated, the investigators concluded that antiandrogen therapy seems to be beneficial in the treatment of HS. The study was limited because of unjustified sample size and no intention-to-treat analysis.

Surgery

For surgical procedures for HS there is a lack of RCTs.[25] Buimer and colleagues[17] conducted a nonblinded randomized study to investigate whether enclosure of antibiotics after primary excision and closure reduces the number of postoperative complications. A total of 200 patients was included, of whom 76 patients were treated with excision and primary closure only, and 124 patients received an additional 5 × 5 cm gentamicin-collagen sponge after surgery. Overall, 59% of the patients treated with gentamicin had no complications, like dehiscence and infection, after 1 week, versus 47% in the group without antibiotics (*P*<.03). However, this significant difference was not seen after 3 months. Also, gentamicin had no significant influence on the local recurrence rate and the duration of wound healing. Side effects of gentamicin were not reported. Also, no clear assessment of baseline severity was available. The baseline randomization imbalance was caused by early cessation of the study. Although the beneficial effect of gentamicin does not influence the long-term prognosis of HS, the investigators recommend the use of gentamicin after excision.

Laser

Three studies assessed the efficacy of laser treatment, including 1 study on neodymium:yttrium-aluminum-garnet (Nd:YAG) laser treatment and 2 studies concerning intense pulsed light (IPL).[18,21,23,26] Mahmoud and colleagues[18] conducted a randomized, right-left within-patient controlled trial in 22 patients. Patients were treated monthly for 4 months with the Nd:YAG laser and topical treatment consisting of clindamycin 1% lotion and benzoyl peroxide 10% wash. The same topical treatment was applied on the control side of the body. To assess efficacy, a modified scoring system was used, based on Sartorius score, with additional patients' symptoms, including erythema, edema, pain, and discharge. The percentage decrease of severity from baseline, indicating improvement, after 6 months was −72.7% on the laser treated side, and −22.9%

on the control side (P<.001). The treatment was associated with minimal patient discomfort, and 60% of the patients did not experience pain related to laser treatment. There was no clear report on side effects. The suggested mechanism of action of the Nd:YAG laser is destruction of the follicular unit.

Highton and colleagues[21] investigated 18 patients in a within-patient study to determine whether IPL is an effective treatment of HS. One side of the body was treated with IPL, twice a week, for 4 weeks. The contralateral side received no treatment. A significant improvement was seen in Sartorius score averaged for all treated sites compared with baseline, which was maintained at 12 months (−33% vs +3%, P<.001). There was a possible trend toward recurrence at 12 months.

Fadel and Tawfik[23] treated 10 patients in a randomized split-body study to evaluate the efficacy of methylene blue (MB) as a photosensitizer delivered as a niosomal gel and activated by IPL (630 nm). One side of the body was treated with niosomal MB gel and the other side with free MB gel. Patients were treated twice a month, for a maximum of 6 months. The follow-up period was up to 6 months after the last treatment. Treatment efficacy was based on the Sartorius score. A significant difference in reduction of lesions was found: 77.3% for the niosomal MB gel side and 44.1% for the free MB gel side (P>.01). The investigators concluded that the use of niosomal gel as a delivery system for MB provides a better penetration to the deeper layers of the dermis. No side effects occurred.

RANDOMIZED CONTROLLED TRIALS RECENTLY COMPLETED AND ONGOING

Several RCTs have recently been completed or are registered as ongoing and results are awaited.[27]

Biologics

PIONEER I and II, two phase 3, double-blind, randomized, placebo-controlled trials to assess the efficacy and safety of adalimumab, were recently completed. Results have already been partially presented in congresses, and these preliminary reports support the validity of the phase 2 trial reported by Kimball and colleagues.[11] Furthermore, an ongoing randomized, double-blind, controlled trial is registered in order to study the efficacy and safety of anakinra, a human interleukin (IL)-1 receptor antagonist, 100 mg daily for 12 weeks compared with placebo, for the treatment of Hurley stage II and III HS. A phase IIa randomized, double-blind, placebo-controlled, multicenter study to assess the safety, tolerability, and preliminary efficacy of MEDI8968, an blocking antibody to IL-1RI, in patients with moderate to severe HS is registered, with active treatment being given as subcutaneous injection at baseline, week 4, and week 8.

Other Treatments

A prospective RCT comparing the efficacy of carbon dioxide laser excision with surgical deroofing in the treatment of HS is registered. A randomized controlled, single-blind trial comparing efficacy of antibiotic therapy (clindamycin 300 mg twice daily and rifampin 300 mg twice daily for 10 weeks) alone with antibiotic therapy (clindamycin 300 mg twice daily and rifampin 300 mg twice daily for 2 weeks) plus 3 Nd:YAG laser sessions is also registered. In addition, a prospective multicenter blinded RCT comparing the efficacy of povidone topical cream twice daily with 10% benzoyl peroxide topical body wash twice daily for the treatment of HS is currently being conducted.

SUMMARY AND RECOMMENDATIONS

This article emphasizes the need for the use of validated and uniform outcomes in order to facilitate indirect comparison of available treatments and to promote evidence-based clinical practice. HiSCR is a validated outcome that is highly recommended to be used in the future as the primary outcome for assessing the efficacy of antiinflammatory treatments.[12] Future studies should also include a justified sample size, with the use of HiSCR, and a thorough report of side effects, both physician and patient rated (pain, tolerability).

Because HS is a chronic debilitating diseases that leads to low quality of life, working disability, and pain, and that is associated with a high rate of several cardiovascular disease risk factors, future clinical trials should include patient-rated outcomes, especially regarding quality of life, working ability, pain scores, and patient satisfaction. The assessment of the possible effects of various treatments in cardiovascular disease risk factors is also interesting.

Combination of the various available treatment modalities, especially combination of surgical approaches with antiinflammatory treatments (**Fig. 4**), is important. Results from Mahmoud and colleagues[18] provide initial evidence that such a combination can have a positive effect. Adjuvant therapy with topical (clindamycin) or systemic antibiotics and/or TNF inhibitors before surgery may lead to less invasive surgery and better short-term and long-term outcomes in Hurley II and III stages

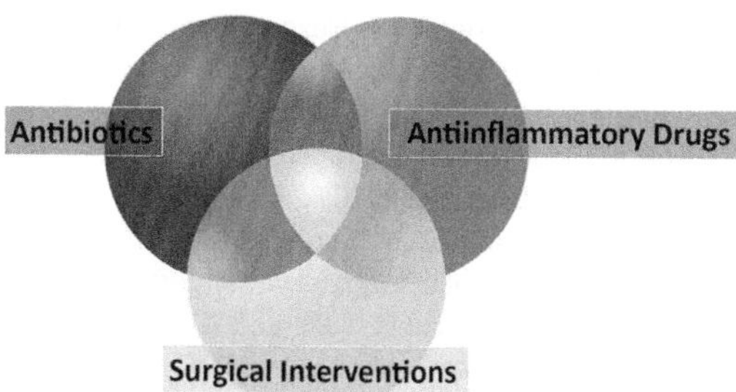

Fig. 4. Combining several treatment options for HS.

of HS. This hypothesis is interesting and warrants further investigation.

Regarding biologics, further evaluation of etanercept is not recommended. Infliximab shows evidence of efficacy, and a possible future clinical trial, with appropriate design and use of validated outcomes, may yield significant results.

HS can be seen at prepubertal ages, with only 2% of cases occurring before the age of 11 years.[28] Data regarding HS in children and adolescents are scarce. So far, recommendations for treating children are based on clinical case reports and extrapolation of the results in adult populations. Randomized multicenter clinical trials with adequate sample sizes are needed to provide high-quality evidence in this specific age group.

The balance between desirable and undesirable outcomes of alternative treatment strategies (the benefit/risk ratio, preferably analyzed with a structured approach) is becoming more and more important, both for treating physicians and for authorities during drug regulatory decision making.[29,30] Future studies should facilitate such assessments. Most of the trials included in this article lack a medium-term and long-term assessment of the efficacy and safety of the studied treatments; future studies should include these assessments.

Implications for Daily Clinical Practice

This article provides evidence that can be used to promote evidence-based daily clinical practice.

For Hurley stage I and mild, not widespread, Hurley II, topical clindamycin 1% solution/gel twice a day for 12 weeks is recommended. Tetracycline 500 by mouth twice a day for 4 months is recommended for more widespread disease. If a patient fails to respond, adalimumab 160 mg subcutaneously at week 0, 80 mg at week 2, then 40 mg weekly, or infliximab (5 mg/kg) intravenously on weeks 0, 2, and 6, and then every 8 weeks can be considered for moderate to severe disease. Hormonal therapy can be considered for moderate to severe disease, especially in women with endocrinologic comorbidities, but the balance between benefits and possible side effects of long-term treatment has to be carefully evaluated. IPL for Hurley II and III stages is also an evidence-based treatment and the use of niosomal MB seems to enhance efficacy. For these stages, Nd:YAG laser monthly for 4 months combined with topical antiinflammatory treatments seems to be a therapeutic option. After surgical excision, addition of local treatments, like a gentamicin-collagen sponge, has been shown to result in fewer complications and is a rational decision.

Integrating Results of Randomized Controlled Trials in the Current State-of-the-art Treatment of Hidradenitis Suppurativa

This article focuses on RCTs only. Hence, several established treatment options are not discussed. According to most experts, the mainstay of treatment in HS is surgical intervention in an early stage of disease, but RCTs on surgical interventions are lacking, probably because it is considered unethical to deny the control group access to surgical treatment for a prolonged period of time. The results of surgery are usually described in prospective or retrospective cohort studies with the percentage of successfully removed lesions as primary outcome. Besides tetracycline, there are other antibiotics that may be even more effective in HS, such as the combination of clindamycin and rifampicin, or clindamycin as monotherapy, but they have not been investigated in RCTs. Most of the recently performed RCTs investigate biologics, and some of these studies are of high quality because they are designed for registration purposes. Antiinflammatory agents reduce inflammation, pain, swelling, and purulent discharge, but epithelialized cavities and fistulas do not disappear. In daily practice, the new antiinflammatory agents are used in combination with other treatment options, as shown in **Fig. 4**. Some patients can be cured with surgery only, some with antibiotics only, and the severe cases may require all treatment modalities, including antiinflammatory agents.

REFERENCES

1. Kurzen H, Kurokawa I, Jemec GB, et al. What causes hidradenitis suppurativa? Exp Dermatol 2008;17:455–72.
2. Jemec GBE. Clinical practice: hidradenitis suppurativa. N Engl J Med 2012;366:158–64.
3. Fimmel S, Zouboulis CC. Comorbidities of hidradenitis suppurativa (acne inversa). Dermatoendocrinol 2010;2:9–16.

4. Esmann S, Jemec GBE. Psychosocial impact of hidradenitis suppurativa: a qualitative study. Acta Derm Venereol 2011;91:328–32.
5. Miller IM, Hamzawi I. Prevalence, risk factors and co-morbidities of hidradenitis suppurativa. Dermatol Clin, in press.
6. Revuz JE, Canoui-Poitrine F, Wolkenstein P, et al. Prevalence and factors associated with hidradenitis suppurativa: results from two case-control studies. J Am Acad Dermatol 2008;59:596–601.
7. Miller IM, Ellervik C, Vinding GR, et al. Association of metabolic syndrome and hidradenitis suppurativa. JAMA Dermatol 2014;150:1273–80.
8. Hurley HJ. Axillary hyperhidrosis, apocrine bromhidrosis, hidradenitis suppurativa, and familial benign pemphigus: surgical approach. In: Roenigk RK, Roenigk HH, editors. Dermatologic surgery. New York: Marcel Dekker; 1996. p. 623–45.
9. Sartorius K, Emtestam L, Jemec GB, et al. Objective scoring of hidradenitis suppurativa reflecting the role of tobacco smoking and obesity. Br J Dermatol 2009;161:831–9.
10. Revuz J, Jemec GBE. Diagnosing hidradentitis suppurativa. Dermatol Clin, in press.
11. Kimball AB, Kerdel F, Adams D, et al. Adalimumab for the treatment of moderate to severe hidradenitis suppurativa: a parallel randomized trial. Ann Intern Med 2012;157:846–55.
12. Kimball AB, Jemec GB, Yang M, et al. Assessing the validity, responsiveness and meaningfulness of the hidradenitis suppurativa clinical response (HiSCR) as the clinical endpoint for hidradenitis suppurativa treatment. Br J Dermatol 2014;171:1434–42.
13. Higgins JPT, Green S, editors. Cochrane handbook for systematic reviews of interventions version 5.1.0 [updated March 2011]. The Cochrane Collaboration. 2011. Available at: www.cochrane-handbook.org. Accessed March 01, 2015.
14. Clemmensen OJ. Topical treatment of hidradenitis suppurativa with clindamycin. Int J Dermatol 1983;22:325–8.
15. Mortimer PS, Dawber RP, Gales MA, et al. A double-blind controlled cross-over trial of cyproterone acetate in females with hidradenitis suppurativa. Br J Dermatol 1986;115:263–8.
16. Jemec GB, Wendelboe P. Topical clindamycin versus systemic tetracycline in the treatment of hidradenitis suppurativa. J Am Acad Dermatol 1998;39:971–4.
17. Buimer MG, Ankersmit MF, Wobbes T, et al. Surgical treatment of hidradenitis suppurativa with gentamicin sulfate: a prospective randomized study. Dermatol Surg 2008;34:224–7.
18. Mahmoud BH, Tierney E, Hexsel CL, et al. Prospective controlled clinical and histopathologic study of hidradenitis suppurativa treated with the long-pulsed neodymium:yttrium-aluminium-garnet laser. J Am Acad Dermatol 2010;62:637–45.
19. Adams DR, Yankura JA, Fogelberg AC, et al. Treatment of hidradenitis suppurativa with etanercept injection. Arch Dermatol 2010;146:501–4.
20. Grant A, Gonzalez T, Montgomery MO, et al. Infliximab therapy for patients with moderate to severe hidradenitis suppurativa: a randomized, double-blind, placebo-controlled crossover trial. J Am Acad Dermatol 2010;62:205–17.
21. Highton L, Chan WY, Khwaja N, et al. Treatment of hidradenitis suppurativa with intense pulsed light: a prospective study. Plast Reconstr Surg 2011;128:459–65.
22. Miller I, Lynggaard CD, Lophaven S, et al. A double-blind placebo-controlled randomized trial of adalimumab in the treatment of hidradenitis suppurativa. Br J Dermatol 2011;165:391–8.
23. Fadel MA, Tawfik AA. New topical photodynamic therapy for treatment of hidradenitis suppurativa using methylene blue niosomal gel: a single-blind, randomized, comparative study. Clin Exp Dermatol 2015;40(2):116–22.
24. Kimball AB, Jemec GBE, Gu Y, et al. A novel hidradenitis suppurativa efficacy variable, HiSCR (Hidradenitis Suppurativa Clinical Response), is responsive to change with adalimumab therapy: results of a phase 2 study. Presented at the 71st Annual Meeting of the American Academy of Dermatology. P6661. Miami Beach, March 1-5, 2013.
25. Horvath B, Mathusiak L. Surgical interventions in hidradentitis suppurativa. Dermatol Clin, in press.
26. Saunte DM, Lapins J. Laser and IPL in hidradentitis suppurativa. Dermatol Clin, in press.
27. Clinical Trial Register of the of the US National Institutes of Health. Available at: http://clinicaltrials.gov. Accessed March 08, 2015.
28. Palmer RA, Keefe M. Early-onset hidradenitis suppurativa. Clin Exp Dermatol 2001;26:501–3.
29. Andrews JC, Schünemann HJ, Oxman AD, et al. GRADE guidelines: 15. Going from evidence to recommendation–determinants of a recommendation's direction and strength. J Clin Epidemiol 2013;66:726–35.
30. US Food and Drug Administration. Structured approach to benefit-risk assessment in drug regulatory decision-making. Available at: http://www.fda.gov/downloads/ForIndustry/UserFees/PrescriptionDrugUserFee/UCM329758.pdf. Accessed December 16, 2014.

Antibiotic Treatment of Hidradenitis Suppurativa

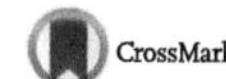

Vincenzo Bettoli, MD[a,*], Olivier Join-Lambert, MD, PhD[b], Aude Nassif, MD[c]

KEYWORDS

• Hidradenitis suppurativa • Antibiotherapy • Antimicrobial resistance • Microbiome-host disease • Acne inversa

KEY POINTS

- Targeted systemic antibiotherapy can dramatically improve hidradenitis suppurativa (HS) but randomized controlled trials are lacking to recommend these treatments.
- Emergence of antibiotic resistance is a major concern.
- Empiric antibiotherapy for HS should target a broad spectrum, including anaerobes; carefully avoid underdosing; and rapidly stop treatment in case of lack of efficacy.
- Clinical remission can be obtained in patients with Hurley stage 1 HS using oral antibiotics (clindamycin-rifampin or rifampin-moxifloxacin-metronidazole) combinations and short-lasting remission or improvement in stage 2 and 3 with intravenous antibiotics. However, in the absence of a validated maintenance treatment, relapses are the rule, indicating the need for a combined antibiotic-surgical treatment.
- A multidisciplinary team including dermatologists, infectious diseases physicians, microbiologists, and surgeons is required to optimize the care of these patients.

Although the pathogenesis of inflammation in hidradenitis suppurativa (HS) is not fully understood, different types of antibiotics (ABs; tetracyclines, rifampin, clindamycin) are widely and increasingly used to treat HS in the absence of validated efficacy data. Considering the prevalence of HS, this issue is critical because potential antimicrobial resistance may hamper the efficacy of ABs and induce comorbidities associated with altered commensal microflora.

RATIONALE/BACKGROUND

- The constant and typical clinical features that define an active HS disease are abscesses, which are also a classic sign of an infectious process.
- Specific ABs are effective in HS.
- In a so-called inflammatory disease, the lack of reports on the efficacy of nonsteroidal antiinflammatory drugs (NSAIDs) and steroids, which are typical antiinflammatory drugs, is surprising and suggests that this disease may be not purely inflammatory.
- Some ABs definitely known to lack an antiinflammatory action (ertapenem, ceftriaxone) are effective in HS. Ertapenem is a β-lactam antibiotic inducing bacterial lysis and thus promoting inflammation. In addition, imipenem, a carbapenem, is considered an

---

Conflicts of Interest: Abbvie, Bioderma, Biogena, Difa-Cooper, Galderma, GSK, L'Oreal, Meda, Pierre-Fabre, Pharcos (V. Bettoli). MSD, Pfizer (O. Join-Lambert). MSD (A. Nassif).

[a] Department of Clinical and Experimental Medicine, OU of Dermatology, Azienda Ospedaliera – University of Ferrara, Via Aldo Moro 8, Località Cona, Ferrara 44100, Italy; [b] Department of Microbiology, INSERM UMR 1151, Team 11 Necker Enfants-Malades Hospital, 149, rue de Sèvres, Paris 75015, France; [c] Medical Center, Institut Pasteur, 25 rue du Dr Roux, Paris 75015, France

* Corresponding author.

E-mail address: vincenzo.bettoli@gmail.com

Dermatol Clin 34 (2016) 81–89

http://dx.doi.org/10.1016/j.det.2015.08.013

0733-8635/16/$ – see front matter

immunoenhancing antibiotic that increases leukocyte chemotaxis and has no antiinflammatory activity.[1]

- In a microbiological study, prolonged cultures saved for 2 weeks were obtained by deep HS lesion biopsies, guided with ultrasonography in order to avoid surface contamination and by swab specimens, and in 4 to 7 days isolated a commensal flora, mostly anaerobic, varying with Hurley severity staging[2] (detailed information is provided elsewhere in this issue). This study may explain the previous results in the literature: sterile because of a too-short length of culture, variable because of a rich commensal flora, and delay in growing depending on the species. These results also question the relevance and pathogenicity of this commensal flora in HS. However, if this flora is considered opportunistic in a genetically predisposed individual, this may explain the failures of ABs when they are not targeted against the isolated flora and also when the length of treatment is too short to eliminate bacteria in a host who has an innate immune anomaly, not allowing the clearance of these germs in the usual length of time.

CLINICAL STUDIES: REVIEW

Methods

A search was performed on PubMed using the terms "hidradenitis suppurativa" or "acne inversa" and "antibiotics," from 1950 to 2015. Excluding randomized controlled trials (RCTs), which are described elsewhere in this issue, studies including at least 10 patients were retained.[3–8] Minor studies with fewer than 10 patients were also reviewed but are briefly mentioned here. Studies using concomitant oral or topical non-AB medications were excluded.

Parameters studied were design and objectives (improvement vs remission), number of patients, outcome with mode of clinical assessment (clinical score of severity used), length of follow-up, initial severity, and side effects. Results are summarized in **Table 1**.

Results

Major studies analyzed in the table concern only systemic ABs.[3–8]

Four studies are focused on the oral combination of rifampin and clindamycin.[3–6] All 4 are case series with a total of 187 patients included and 128 who concluded the studies. Three are retrospective evaluations, whereas only 1 is prospective and none is a RCT. The dosage is usually 600 mg daily for both ABs and the duration is 10 weeks in most cases, except for 1 study with different dosages and duration.[3] The most frequently considered outcome measures are Sartorius and Hurley scores, whereas number of outbreaks, Patient Global Assessment (PGA) and Physician Global Assessment (PhGA), quality of life, pain, and suppuration scores are less frequently calculated.

The combination of both ABs obtained good clinical efficacy in 71% to 93% of the cases. Parameters used included Sartorius improvement greater than 25% in 1 study and statistically significant in another, Hurley reduction of at least 1 stage, PhGA partial improvement less than 75%, and total improvement greater than 75%. In 1 study the outcome measure was not reported. No difference in terms of response with 5 different dosages was reported in 1 study.[3] Positive clinical results might also be obtained with treatment duration shorter than 10 weeks.[3] Continuing the treatment in non responders over 10 weeks did not bring any beneficial effect.

Side effects were reported in 13% to 38% of the patients. Gastrointestinal side effects were most frequently reported. The treatment was stopped in 4% to 26% of the cases. *Clostridium difficile* colitis does not seem to be a significant side effect with this treatment, since no case was reported in these 4 studies.

Only 1 of the 4 studies reported data on the follow-up.[4] Eight patients out of the 13 who were followed up (61%) showed a relapse of the disease after a mean duration of 5 months.

However, a new treatment may not be as beneficial as the first one in the same patient, questioning the role of an acquired resistance to this combination. A possible explanation for this secondary resistance is the liver enzymatic induction by rifampin, acting as a major inducer of cytochrome P450 3A4, the main metabolic pathway of clindamycin. This enzymatic induction may significantly reduce the plasma concentration of orally taken clindamycin and result in resistance to clindamycin and rifampin caused by the use of a monotherapy of rifampin, which is well known to be highly mutagenic.[9]

Another study evaluated the efficacy of intravenous (IV) ertapenem in 30 cases of Hurley II and III HS. After 6 weeks, 17 out of 30 patients improved by at least 1 point in the Hurley scale.[7] A dramatic improvement was observed in very severe cases, although this antibiotic has no recognized antiinflammatory activity. However, the structure of the study (a case series, retrospective, without a control group, and with no follow-up) has important limitations.

The oral combination of rifampin plus moxifloxacin plus metronidazole provided clinical remission (disappearance of pain, draining, and erythema, as well as softening of hypertrophic scars in all the involved areas) in all Hurley I cases (6 out of 6) in a mean time of 2.4 months, 8 out of 10 Hurley II cases in a mean time of 3.8 months, and 2 out of 12 Hurley III cases in 6.2 and 12 months[8] Lack of control group, wide variability in severity, and length of treatment limit the value of the data but the positive role of ABs in HS is again implied.

Another study concerned 24 patients using dapsone in a retrospective review of open case series.[10] An improvement was observed in 9 out of 24 (38%) patients. No improvement was seen in the remaining 15 patients, including 4 severe cases. Side effects leading to suspension of the treatment occurred in 2 out of 24 (8%) patients. Recurrence came quickly after stopping. This finding suggests that dapsone may find an indication in mild cases of HS.

A different study assessed retrospective efficacy of AB only in general and not of a specific AB strategy in a cohort of 115 patients with HS: this retrospective evaluation yielded an 80% rate of improvement with ABs.[11]

One important bias in all these studies is the lack of information on the possible concurrent stopping of NSAIDs and/or steroids during treatment and diabetes management optimization. In the experience of one of the authors, all these measures may significantly improve the disease and may suppress flares in mild forms of HS.

Studies concerning single cases or fewer than 10 patients have occasionally reported improvement or remission in separate patients with AB, mainly minocycline or dapsone, but these studies often concern a combination of concomitant treatments (isotretinoin, cyproterone acetate, biotherapies, and/or immune-suppressive drugs), making assessment of only the AB used in the combination impossible. Therefore, these cases have not been included in this article.

In about 25% of histologic samples of patients with HS, foreign body–type granulomas are found.[12] Isoniazid is an antituberculosis drug with antibacterial and antigranulomatous effects. It has been used at the dosage of 300 mg daily for 3 months in an open study including 4 patients with HS, Hurley II or III stage. The results did not indicate any beneficial effect.[13]

A study reported remission in 4 patients with HS (Hurley II) treated with broad-spectrum ABs, including ertapenem IV, and an association of IV ceftriaxone and oral metronidazole as induction treatment.[14] Broad-spectrum IV ABs may therefore induce complete remission even in patients with severe HS. IV administration of ABs should be considered in severe cases, and issues of resistance not neglected.

One patient with a severe Hurley III HS was put into remission with 1.2 g of linezolid and meropenem 1 g IV daily for 1 month, which are also ABs not known to have any antiinflammatory activity.[15] Two weeks later a relapse developed, questioning the importance of a maintenance treatment or of surgery to remove residual biofilms, which can be a constant source of relapse in HS scars.

However, lack of RCTs and heterogeneity of the populations, mostly in terms of severity and different outcome measures, do not allow detailed and definite conclusions to be drawn.

GENERAL RULES FOR ANTIBIOTIC USE

Routes of Administration

- Topical applications may be attractive for a dermatologic disease because of direct action on the targeted organ (skin) without unwanted systemic side effects. However, clinicians should keep in mind that HS lesions are usually deep and thick, so a purely topical treatment may not penetrate deep enough to reach lesions or the entire lesion, and the level of absorption through a scarred skin may be variable.
- Systemic administrations include oral, intramuscular (IM), and IV (IV) routes.

For the oral route, clinicians should take into account:

- Absorption problems, especially those caused by IBD because they can be associated with HS (discussed elsewhere in this issue).
- Elimination problems caused by renal insufficiency, which necessitate an adaptation of dosages for all routes of administration.
- Contraindications should be respected: for example, rifampin should not be prescribed in a patient presenting chronic hepatitis, and moxifloxacin cannot be prescribed in individuals with cardiac rythm and/or conduction anomalies (an electrocardiogram is mandatory before prescribing moxifloxacin).
- Physicians should also be aware of potential interactions of ABs with other medications prescribed for associated diseases. For instance, rifampin is an inducer of cytochrome P450 and may dramatically decrease the blood level of not only the contraceptive pill but also antiepileptic and kidney transplant immune-suppressive drugs, so blood levels of these drugs should be carefully monitored.

IM or IV administration may be a good option in moderate to severe patients for ABs that have no oral forms. The advantages are 100% compliance

Table 1
Results of main clinical studies of AB in HS

Study	Aim of the Study	Type of Study	Patients/Treatment	Outcome Measures	Results	Side Effects	Limitations	Follow-up
Systemic AB								
Bettoli et al,[3] 2014	• Assess efficacy and tolerance: rifampin + clindamycin • Severe, actively inflammatory cases	• Prospective • Noncomparative • Case series	pts: 23 (16 F, 7 M) do: clindamycin 600 mg; rifampin 600 mg du: 10 wk	Sartorius: r = improvement >25% reduction of flare-up	sc: 20 of 23 re: 17 of 20 (85%) dro[b]: 3 of 23 Sartorius mean reduction: 45% Flare-up: mean reduction: 60%	se: 3 of 23 (13%), mostly nausea and vomiting st: 1 of 3	No randomization No control group	No
Nassif et al,[7] 2012	• Evaluate efficacy and tolerance • Ertapenem 1 g IV • Severe HS	• Retrospective • Case series	pts: 30 Hurley: II, 18 pts; III, 12 pts do: ertapenem 1 g IV daily du: 6 wk	Hurley: r = reduction of at least 1 stage	Hurley: re = 17 of 30 8 pts (III>II) 8 pts (II>I) 1 pt (II>0) 13 of 30 pts (unchanged)	se: • 9 of 29 pts headaches • 8 of 29 pts candidiasis	No randomization No control group Retrospective	No
Join-Lambert et al,[8] 2011	• Assess efficacy and safety • Rifampin, moxifloxacin, metronidazole • Long-lasting cases refractory to previous treatments	• Retrospective • Case series • Consecutive patients • Included in a short period of time	pts: 28 (20 F, 8 M) Hurley I (6) Hurley II (10) Hurley III (12) do: metronidazole 1.5 g/d Rifampin 10 mg/kg/d Moxifloxacin 400 mg/d du: 4–6 wk; possible repeated courses	cr: clearance of all inflammatory lesions including hypertrophic scars	cr: 16 of 28 Hurley I: 6 of 6 (2.4[a]) Hurley II: 8 of 10 (3.8 m[a]) Hurley III: 2 of 12 (6.2 m[a] first pt) (12 m[a] second pt)	se: GI disorders (64%) Vaginal candidiasis (35% of F)	No randomization No control group Different length of treatment Pretreatment with IV ceftriaxone and oral metronidazole in 14 patients Different severities Retrospective	Follow-up on: 14 of 16 cr Duration: 2–12 mo Secondary prophylaxis: 13 of 14 (TMP-SMZ 12 pts) or doxycycline (1 pt) Relapse: 7 of 14

Van der Zee et al,[4] 2009	Expand and validate the basis of the combination clindamycin + rifampin	• Retrospective • Case series	pts: treated, 47; assessed, 34 5 different dosages, details not specified 23 of 34 do: rifampin 600 mg, clindamycin 600 mg du: 10 wk	Hurley Physician GA pi: <75% ti: >75%	re: 28 of 34 (82%) pi: 12 of 28 (35%) ti: 16 of 28 (47%) nr: 6 of 34 (18%) Length of treatment: No difference among: 10 wk, >10 wk, <10 wk High percentage of nonresponders in group 10 wk or longer No predominant response in severe cases	se: 13 of 34 (38%) 9 of 13 diarrhea 9 of 34 (26%) stopped for side effects 6 of 9 (diarrhea) No cases positive for *Clostridium difficile* colitis	No randomization No control group Different severities Heterogeneity of the included groups and few patients each group Retrospective	13 of 34 Relapse 8 of 13 (61%) After 5.0 mo (mean)
Gener et al,[5] 2009	Evaluate efficacy Clindamycin + rifampin Different severity (Hurley I, II, III)	• Retrospective • Case series • Consecutive patients	pts treated: 116 pts analyzed: 70 do: clindamycin 600 mg + rifampin 600 mg du: 10 wk	Sartorius: improvement statistically significant Hurley Pain and Suppuration score (numerical scale 0–10) QoL score Patient GA	pts: 70 cr: 8 of 70 (11%) si: 59 of 70 (82%) nr: 1 of 70 w: 2 of 70 Pain score (7>3) Suppuration score (6>2)	se: 10 of 70 nausea, diarrhea, abdominal pain 1 of 10 skin eruption st: 8 of 10	No randomization No control group Different severities Decision to treat on clinical ground	No
Mendonca et al,[6] 2006	Assess efficacy: clindamycin and rifampin	• Retrospective • Case series	pts: 14 (9 F, 5 M) do: clindamycin 600 mg Rifampin 600 mg du: 10 wk	Complete remission (parameter not detailed)	cr: 10 of 14 (71%) (8 rifampin/ clindamycin 2 rifampin/ minocycline)	se: 6 of 14 diarrhea 2 of 6 clindamycin > minocycline 4 of 6 dro	No randomization No control group Retrospective No data on disease severity	

Abbreviations: cr, complete remission; do, dosage; dro, drop out; du, duration; GI, gastrointestinal; IV, intravenous; nr, no response; pi, partial improvement; pts, patients; QoL, quality of life; r, responsivity; re, responders; sc, study completed; se, side effects; si, significant improvement; st, stop treatment; ti, total improvement; TMP-SMZ, trimethoprim/sulfamethoxazole; w, worse.

[a] Patients who met the responsivity criteria.

[b] Flare-up = exacerbation of a single lesion (inflammation / discharge of purulent material).

(a nurse performing the IM injections or infusions daily at home), a better diffusion into scarred tissue without the problem of intestinal absorption and of the liver metabolic barrier, no gastrointestinal side effects, and the rapidity of the IM injection procedure. Disadvantages include pain caused by IM injections, which usually prevents a use for more than 3 weeks, and, for IV infusions, the length of the procedure (usually a half hour for a daily infusion).

The IV route may be mandatory for ABs that have no other mode of administration. These usually potent ABs with broad spectra should be reserved for very severe patients at Hurley 3, who usually justify a prolonged IV treatment of at least 6 weeks, in order to restore a quality of life and make surgery possible in patients considered otherwise inoperable. For those selected severe cases, a peripherally inserted central catheter should be inserted during a 1-day hospitalization. The advantage of this catheter is its easiness to insert and use, but, as with any catheter, thrombosis and infection, although rare, may occur.

Side Effects

Potential side effects observed with ABs are numerous and should always be taken into account before any prescription of an AB, as well as possible interactions with the patient's own treatments. Unwanted effects can be divided into short-term effects and long-term effects.

Short-term side effects

These usually regress after stopping the medication and can be subdivided into side effects common to all the ABs and those specific of a class of AB.

Common to all antibiotics

- Oral, digestive, vaginal, and/or skin candidiasis should be looked for at each visit when patients are under ABs and can easily be taken care of with topical or oral antifungals.
- Allergy: urticaria, Quincke edema, acute generalized pustulosis (AGEP), exanthematous drug rash, stevens-johnson syndrome (SJS), toxic epidermal necrosis (TEN), drug reaction eosinophilia and systemic syndrome (DRESS) syndrome, fixed drug eruption can potentially be observed with many ABs.

Specific to 1 class of antibiotics These should be searched for at each visit according to the AB prescribed (**Table 2**) and prevented as far as possible (eg, avoid sport with quinolones; stop metronidazole and linezolid after 6 consecutive weeks to avoid neuropathy; wear sunscreen in case of sun

Table 2
Antibiotic side effects

Antibiotic	Side Effects
Rifampin	Hepatitis, pharmacokinetic interaction with drugs metabolized in the liver via cytochrome P450 activation (inefficacy of oral contraception), nausea, diarrhea, rare hematologic disorders and rare joint pain, orange coloration of urine
Clindamycin	*C difficile* infections (pseudomembranous colitis), nausea, vomiting, diarrhea, abdominal pain, rare hematologic disorders
Cyclins	Abdominal pain, esophagitis, diarrhea, phototoxicity (doxycycline)
Metronidazole	Peripheral neuropathy (with consecutive use >6 wk), vertigo, asthenia, depression, general malaise, hematologic (leucopenia), dysgeusia, abdominal pain, nausea, vomiting, diarrhea
Moxifloxacin	Tendon rupture, photosensitivity
β-Lactams: amoxicillin, amoxicillin + clavulanic acid, ceftriaxone, ertapenem	Gastrointestinal
Co-trimoxazole	Hematologic (anemia, leucopenia)
Dapsone	Hemolytic anemia with methemoglobinemia
Linezolid	Thrombopenia (usually after 10 d of treatment), leucopenia, anemia, peripheral neuropathy (for long-term use); linezolid should not be prescribed for more than 6 wk

exposure under doxycycline and quinolones; monitor liver enzymes with rifampin; monitor white cell count with co-trimoxazole; monitor platelet count with linezolid).

Long-term side effects (risk of resistance)

- In individuals who are treated for skin, leading to lack of efficacy for HS, and also in other organs, including intestinal microbiota with a risk of secondary resistance for other illnesses.
- In the general population: knowing the prevalence of HS, this is a major concern in the long term. Without understanding this risk, AB use could be very deleterious not only for the individuals treated but for the population.

Rules to limit emergence of resistance:

- Prescriptions of ABs should be reserved for patients who are seriously affected by the disease.
- Avoid underdosages.
- Do not prescribe ABs if the patient is not adherent to the prescribed therapy, leading to an irregular and incomplete treatment that promotes the acquisition of bacterial resistance.
- Reserve broad-spectrum ABs for severely ill patients for induction treatment and for a limited time with an ultimate surgical objective.
- Plan surgery after cooling the lesions in cases of more than 2 consecutive relapses in the same scar within 6 months. This approach avoids the regular use of ABs for relapses.
- Relapses in scars after a clinical remission can be secondary to reinfections or inability of ABs to eradicate bacterial persisters. Surgery should then be considered in order to obtain a definitive remission in the involved area and could be optimized with a new antibiotic treatment for 2 to 3 weeks before the excision. Alternatively, other therapies could be proposed.
- For maintenance treatment, use a narrow-spectrum AB, not used in active treatment of HS.

DISCUSSION

Numerous case series and retrospective studies indicate remission or clear improvement of HS with AB treatment, and therefore raise the question of whether the observed effects are caused by an antiinfectious or antiinflammatory mechanism of action for these ABs.

If the mode of action of an AB is primarily antiinflammatory, the prescriber should be conscious that any administration of AB, even from the perspective of an antiinflammatory effect, will expose all the commensal flora of the patient to the AB. In this respect, small dosages inducing resistances should be avoided. All the rules mentioned earlier must be met.

In contrast, if the mode of action is primarily antimicrobial, then the strategy should be to use precisely targeted ABs against the isolated flora and to propose surgery for relapsing lesions after cooling them in order to avoid frequent use of more potent ABs.

Furthermore, the possibility that both mechanisms are involved cannot be excluded.

Also, physicians may disagree about the balance between benefits and risks of the treatment, with some clinicians accepting mild flares and offering no treatment for Hurley stage I patients or only a short treatment of flares, whereas others think that the goal is complete and sustained remission.

According to the strategy adopted, ABs may be used:

- Only for the treatment of flares and/or relapses after remission
- As induction treatment (to induce remission)
- As subsequent maintenance treatment
- To prepare surgery

Relapse treatment could be the same as treatment of the flare; for example, relying on microbial data, either amoxicillin-clavulanic acid 3 g/d for 1 to 3 weeks or pristinamycin 2 to 3 g/d for 2 to 3 weeks, and, in case of failure after a week, add metronidazole 1 to 1.5 g/d for the following 1 - 2 weeks (**Table 3**).

The purpose of the induction treatment is to achieve remission in less severe patients and prepare severe patients for surgery. Depending on the severity of the disease, itself correlated with the richness of flora,[2] this may need a more potent AB.

The purpose of the maintenance treatment is to avoid relapses after remission. Maintenance treatment should have few or no side effects because it is a long-term treatment.

In this respect, it must be kept in mind that stopping the progression of the disease is achievable. A postal follow-up survey reported a remission in 39.4% (50 of 124) of the patients, and this method is much easier in mild to moderate cases when the disease is in the early phases.[16] Also, one of the investigators never observed the occurrence of a new area of involvement (relapses always occur in old scars) under AB in any patient in 8 years of different AB strategies in a cohort of 500 treated patients (personal unpublished data from A Nassif, 2015), or in young patients with new HS disease,

Table 3
Recommendations according to the severity of the disease

Proposed Recommendations According to Severity	Therapeutic Options
Hurley I: Mild, few flares, 3–4 a year; no particular discomfort for the patient	1. No AB treatment 2. Treatment only in case of a flare[a]
Hurley I: Moderate, more than 3–4 flares a year and discomfort for the patient	1. Treatment only in case of a flare[a] 2. Induction oral treatment[b] + maintenance treatment[c]
Hurley II: Moderate to severe	Induction IM or IV treatment[d], then oral consolidation + maintenance treatment[c]
Hurley III	Induction IM or IV treatment[d], then oral consolidation + maintenance treatment[c]

These are propositions based on the daily practice of the authors, but only well-designed RCTs will be able to prove the efficacy of these strategies.

[a] If no results with topical clindamycin and pain killers, and drainage of purulent material not applicable: amoxicillin, amoxicillin plus clavulanic acid 1 g $\times$ 3 for 1 to 3 weeks or pristinamycin 2–3 g/d for 2 to 3 weeks and, in case of failure after 1 week, add metronidazole 1 to 1.5 g/d for 2 weeks.

[b] Rifampin 600 mg/d plus clindamycin 600 mg/d for 10 weeks or the combination rifampin-moxifloxacin-metronidazole for 6 weeks then 4 weeks of rifampin-moxifloxacin. If clindamycin not tolerated: cyclins or oral metronidazole.

[c] Cyclines or dapsone or sulfamethoxazole 400 mg/d (800 mg/d if weight >90 kg).

[d] Ceftriaxone plus metronidazole for 3 weeks then rifampin-moxifloxacin-metronidazole for 3 weeks, then rifampin-moxifloxacin for 6 weeks for Hurley II. Hurley III may benefit from prolonged ertapenem for 6 weeks as induction treatment.

coming from families with Hurley stage 3 disease once they are under AB.

In the absence of prospective controlled trials, validating the use of AB in HS, no recommendation can reasonably be proposed from literature analysis either for induction or maintenance treatment.

However, recommendation for patients who should not be treated with AB may include:

- Nonadherent patients who do not take the treatment regularly, and/or do not perform the necessary checkups for monitoring side effects, and/or cannot come for follow-up visits
- Patients for whom suppressing a triggering factor (eg, diabetes or NSAIDs/steroids) results in disappearance of all the flares after 3 months (personal unpublished data from A Nassif, 2015)

CONCLUSION

A proposition to treat only the flare could be offered to patients with Hurley stage I HS who have fewer than 4 flares a year lasting less than 3 weeks, but because there is no validated treatment of a common flare of HS, no recommendation can be outlined from this literature study.

Because no single medical treatment is efficient for curing HS, a strategy to obtain and maintain remission should rely on several treatment modalities in order to avoid prolonged use of potent treatments with potential deleterious side effects. Because HS is a complex and heterogeneous disease that is difficult to treat, a global and multidisciplinary approach to the disease and all its components should be attempted, combining several treatments to obtain remission. ABs should be thought of only as a part of a complete strategy including ablative methods such as surgery and laser, general measures (losing weight for overweighed patients), and eventually immune modulators. The objectives are to relieve symptoms in severely affected patients and to prevent relapses but also to prevent regular use of broad-spectrum ABs, and in this way to avoid the occurrence of resistances. The targeted use of ABs is a mainstay for preparation of HS patients to surgery, since excision is easier when the infectious and inflammatory components of the disease have cooled.[8,9,17]

Even though there are a lot of arguments in favor of a beneficial effect of ABs in HS, these treatments should be used with consideration of the ratio between benefits and risks. There is therefore a great need for scientific assessment and validation of the efficacy and tolerance profiles in the short and long terms for these treatments before clinicians will be able to prescribe them correctly. It is the duty of dermatologists to design appropriate studies to show which ABs can be effective in HS.

REFERENCES

1. Van Vlem B, Vanholder R, De Paepe P, et al. Immunomodulating effects of antibiotics: literature review. Infection 1996;24:275–91.
2. Guet-Revillet H, Coignard-Biehler H, Jais JP, et al. Bacterial pathogens associated with hidradenitis suppurativa. Emerg Infect Dis 2014; 20(12):1990–8.
3. Bettoli V, Zauli S, Borghi A, et al. Oral clindamycin and rifampicin in the treatment of hidradenitis suppurativa – acne inversa: a prospective study on 23 patients. J Eur Acad Dermatol Venereol 2014; 28(1):125–6.
4. van der Zee HH, Boer J, Prens EP, et al. The effects of combined treatment with oral clindamycin and oral rifampicin in patients with hidradenitis suppurativa. Dermatology 2009;14:143–7.
5. Gener G, Canoui-Poitrine F, Revuz JE, et al. Combination therapy with clindamycin and rifampicin for hidradenitis suppurativa: a series of 116 consecutive patients. Dermatology 2009;219:148–54.
6. Mendonca CO, Griffiths CE. Clindamycin and rifampicin combination therapy for hidradenitis suppurativa. Br J Dermatol 2006;154:977–8.
7. Join-Lambert O, Coignard H. Efficacy of IV ertapenem as induction treatment for severe HS. Late Breaking Research Symposium, American Academy of Dermatology Annual Meeting, San Diego, March 16–20, 2012, Communication.
8. Join-Lambert O, Coignard H, Jais JP, et al. Efficacy of rifampin-moxifloxacin-metronidazole combination therapy in hidradenitis suppurativa. Dermatology 2011;222(1):49–58.
9. Join-Lambert O, Ribadeau-Dumas F, Jullien V, et al. Dramatic reduction of clindamycin plasma concentration in hidradenitis suppurativa patients treated with the rifampin-clindamycin combination. Eur J Dermatol 2014;24(1):94–5.
10. Yazdanyar S, Boer J, Ingvarsson G, et al. Dapsone therapy for hidradenitis suppurativa: a series of 24 patients. Dermatology 2011;222(4):342–6.
11. Kohorst JJ, Hagen C, Baum CL, et al. Treatment experience in a local population with hidradenitis suppurativa. J Drugs Dermatol 2014;13(7):827–31.
12. Jemec GB, Hansen U. Histology of hidradenitis suppurativa. J Am Acad Dermatol 1996;34:994–9.
13. Miller IM, Dufour DN, Jemec GB. Treatment of hidradenitis suppurativa: is oral isoniazid an option? J Dermatolog Treat 2012;23:128–30.
14. Nassif A, Coignard-Biehler H, Lortholary O, et al. Complete remission of severe hidradenitis suppurativa obtained in 4 patients using wide spectrum antimicrobial treatment. Academy of Dermatology Annual Meeting, San Diego, March 16–20, 2012, poster n.5181.
15. Scheinfeld N. Extensive hidradenitis suppurativa (HS) Hurley stage III disease treated with intravenous (IV) linezolid and meropenem with rapid remission. Dermatol Online J 2015;21.
16. Kromann CB, Deckers IE, Esmann S, et al. Risk factors, clinical course and long-term prognosis in hidradenitis suppurativa: a cross-sectional study. Br J Dermatol 2014;171(4):819–24.
17. Nesmith RB, Merkel KL, Mast BA. Radical surgical resection combined with lymphadenectomy-directed antimicrobial therapy yielding cure of severe axillary hidradenitis. Ann Plastic Surg 2013; 70:538–41.

Medical Treatments of Hidradenitis Suppurativa

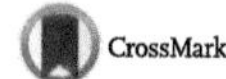

More Options, Less Evidence

Hessel H. van der Zee, MD, PhD[a,*],
Wayne P. Gulliver, BSc, MD, FRCPC, FACP[b]

KEYWORDS

- Hidradenitis suppurativa • Acne inversa • Treatment • Evidence

KEY POINTS

- Very few randomized, control trials are available for the treatment of hidradenitis suppurativa.
- Most therapies reviewed in this article have Category of Evidence IV and Strength of Recommendation D.
- Acitretin, zinc gluconate and metformin have a Category of Evidence III and Strength of Recommendation C.

INTRODUCTION

Hidradenitis suppurativa (HS) is a chronic inflammatory skin disease characterized by painful recurrent nodules and abscesses that often rupture and lead to significant pain with the formation of sinus tracts and scarring. This common disorder (affecting approximately 1% of the population) can be psychologically debilitating and have a significant negative impact on the patient's quality of life.

With the recent publication of Guidelines for HS Treatment, produced by the European Dermatology Forum,[1] as well as recent evidence-based approach to the treatment of HS,[2] we can now develop a comprehensive, holistic, and rational approach to the treatment of this chronic, debilitating, devastating, recurrent inflammatory disorder of the skin. In this article, we review the evidence for many of the second and third line therapies for the treatment of HS. Because very few randomized, controlled trials are available for the treatment of HS, therapies presented are mainly based on case series and case reports. All the therapies reviewed in this article have Category of Evidence IV and Strength of Recommendation D with the exception of acitretin, zinc gluconate, and metformin, which have a Category of Evidence III and Strength of Recommendation C (**Table 1**).

BIOLOGIC THERAPY

Ustekinumab a combined interleukin (IL)-12 and IL-23 inhibitor has also been used in the treatment of HS with a total of 3 case reports. Three patients showed a cumulative response rate of 33% with relapse noted after discontinuation of treatment in 2 of the 3 patients.[3] Recently, an open-label study of 17 patients has been reported and published in an abstract forum.[4] In this unpublished, open-label, prospective study, 35% of patients achieved a meaningful clinical response at week 40 ($\geq$50% improvement in standardized clinical scores). This same study reported greater than 5-point decrease in Dermatology Life Quality Index in 47% of patients.[3] Evidence Category IV, Strength of Recommendation D (see **Table 1**).

[a] Department of Dermatology, Erasmus Medical Center, Burgemeester s' Jacobplein 51, 3015 CA Rotterdam, The Netherlands; [b] Faculty of Medicine, Memorial University of Newfoundland, St. John's, NL A1B 3V6, Canada
* Corresponding author.
E-mail address: h.vanderzee@erasmusmc.nl

Dermatol Clin 34 (2016) 91–96
http://dx.doi.org/10.1016/j.det.2015.08.006

Table 1
Table of evidence for nonrandomized, controlled trial tested treatment options for hidradenitis suppurativa

Therapy	Category of Evidence	Strength of Recommendation
Ustekinumab	IV	D
Steroids (intralesional/ systemic)	IV	D
Dapsone	IV	D
Cyclosporine	IV	D
Hormones	IV	D
Pain control and dressings	IV	D
Isotretinoin	IV	D
Acitretin	III	C
Alitretinoin	IV	D
Resorcinol	IV	D
Gamma-globulin	IV	D
Colchicine	IV	D
Metformin	III	C
Zinc gluconate	III	C
Botulinum toxin	IV	D
Fumarates	IV	D
Tacrolimus	IV	D

STEROIDS, INTRALESIONAL SYSTEMIC

The use of intralesional systemic corticosteroids is the mainstay of rescue therapy in the management of HS. Intralesional triamcinolone acetonide 5 to 10 mg/mL is widely used for the management of acute flares of single or limited number of abscesses.[5] This therapy may also be helpful for the treatment of recalcitrant nodules and sinus tracts.[5] Clinical response is usually rapid within 48 to 72 hours. Well-known adverse events of atrophy, pigmentary changes, and telangiectasia can been seen with intralesional corticosteroid use. This therapy is contraindicated if there is presence of cellulitis. At the recommended doses, systemic side effects are uncommon.[6] Complications are that of superinfection.[6] Evidence Category IV, Strength of Recommendation D (see **Table 1**).

SYSTEMIC CORTICOSTEROIDS

In HS patients with significant flares, systemic corticosteroids may be used as rescue therapy. It is recommended that the dose and duration be minimized to limit the long-term complications of prolonged systemic steroid use. For acute flares, doses equivalent to 0.5 and 0.7 mg/kg of prednisolone may be useful. Therapy should be limited tapering occurring over a few weeks.[7] In addition to systemic steroids being useful for the control of acute flares, the occasional case report of sustained disease control up to 12 months.[7] Long-term treatment with systemic corticosteroids is not currently recommended because of the potential health risk of prolonged steroid use. Evidence Category IV, Strength of Recommendation D (see **Table 1**).

DAPSONE

Dapsone is an antibiotic with marked antiinflammatory properties, especially in neutrophilic dermatosis. The use of dapsone in doses of 50 to 200 mg/d for 1 to 48 months has been reported in retrospective review of 24 patients.[8] Meaningful clinical improvement was observed in 38% of cases. Adverse events were not uncommon and led to withdrawal of therapy in 8%. Rapid relapse of the HS occurred in patients who discontinued therapy. A second but smaller retrospective study reported significant improvement in all 5 cases.[9] Evidence Category IV, Strength of Recommendation D (see **Table 1**).

CYCLOSPORINE

Cyclosporine as monotherapy or in combination with corticosteroids has been reported in only 4 cases. Cyclosporine is a calcineurin inhibitor. It targets T lymphocytes. Doses range from 1 to 6 mg/kg/d. Patients reported to have moderate to sustained response with therapies lasting from 6 weeks to 4 months.[10–12] Because of the significant adverse event profile of cyclosporine, it is recommended that it be used by health care providers with both experience and knowledge in the use of cyclosporine. Evidence Category IV, Strength of Recommendation D (see **Table 1**).

HORMONES

A number of hormone therapies have been reported. Antiandrogen, cyproterone acetate, and ethinyl estradiol have been noted in case series to show improvement in HS. Progesterone has been associated with both the onset of HS as well as worsening of preexisting disease. In a case series of 4 females with longstanding HS a combination of cyproterone acetate 100 mg/d and ethinyl estradiol had controlled the patients HS. Relapse was noted once the dose of cyproterone acetate was lowered to 50 mg/d.[13] Another case series involving females treated with 19 nortestosterone derivatives noted induction or exacerbation of HS. Other types of contraceptives have not been noted to affect the natural history of this disease in this same case series.[14] How hormones influence HS pathogenesis it not known. Evidence Category IV, Strength of Recommendation D (see **Table 1**).

PAIN CONTROL

Because significant pain is a common symptom of HS, its management is a significant aspect of the holistic approach to the treatment of HS.[2] To date, no clinical evidence has been published for the use of nonsteroidal anti-inflammatory drugs in the treatment of pain and inflammation associated with HS. The use of nonsteroidal anti-inflammatory drugs is based on a physician's clinical experience. Evidence Category IV, Strength of Recommendation D (see **Table 1**).

Opiates

Opiates are used commonly for pain control. To date, no studies have been conducted on their use in patients with HS. The use of opiates should be based on a physician's clinical experience and local guidelines. These drugs have significant addictive properties, so short-term use is highly recommended. Evidence Category IV, Strength of Recommendation D (see **Table 1**).

DRESSINGS

As in many of the second- and third-line therapies for the treatment of HS, no randomized controlled trials or cases have been published studying the use of specific dressings or wound care methodology in the treatment of HS.[2] Owing to the lack of clinical evidence the choice of dressing and wound care program implemented by the health care professional has to be based solely on clinical experience. Evidence Category IV, Strength of Recommendation D.

ISOTRETINOIN

The efficacy of isotretinoin has been studied in several case reports and 2 case series.[15–21] Boer and van Gemert[15] studied a group of patients in a retrospective case series of 64 patients with mild to moderate HS. They treated for 4 to 6 months with a mean dose of 0.56 mg/kg. Twenty-nine percent (29%) did not complete the minimum of 4 months treatment. Patients dropped out because a lack of efficacy or adverse side effects. Twenty-four percent of patients achieved clearance. Soria and colleagues[16] interviewed 358 consecutive HS patients regarding the effect of previous treatment with oral isotretinoin. Fourteen patients (16.1%) declared an improvement, 67 patients (77%) no effect, and 6 patients (6.9%) worsening of HS. The authors concluded that oral isotretinoin was not effective in the treatment of HS. The rational for isotretinoin use for the treatment of HS was based on the now outdated opinion that HS has a similar pathogenesis as acne vulgaris. The current opinion is that reduction of sebaceous gland size and inhibition of sebaceous gland activity is not of relevance in HS pathogenesis. Because data are inconsistent and its use in HS is often disappointing, it is recommended not to use isotretinoin in the treatment of HS.[1] Evidence Category IV, Strength of Recommendation D. (see **Table 1**).

ACITRETIN

Several case reports on the use of acitretin/etretinate therapy are published, including 2 case series, 1 retrospective and 1 prospective.[22–26] In 2011, Boer and Nazary[22] published a retrospective study of 12 patients with severe, recalcitrant HS who were treated with acitretin (mean dose, 0.59 mg/kg/d for 9–12 months). Follow-up was up to 4 years. All patients achieved remission and experienced a significant decrease in pain. Moreover, in 9 patients long-lasting improvement was observed. In 2014, Matusiak and colleagues[23] investigated the clinical efficacy of acitretin monotherapy in 17 patients with long-standing and recalcitrant HS in a prospective open-label trial. The patients were treated with acitretin for up to 9 months. The mean acitretin dose was 0.56 mg/kg/d. Nine patients (53%) finished the 9 months of acitretin treatment. A significant improvement was observed after only 1 month of therapy, and further improvement was seen during the next few months. Eight subjects (47%) fulfilled the criteria for response (hidradenitis suppurativa severity index [HSSI] $\geq$ 50% reduction from baseline). However, the dropout rate was high (47%), owing mostly to drug ineffectiveness and adverse events. Discontinuation of treatment resulted in deterioration or relapse of HS 2 to 8 months after acitretin cessation, in all but 1 patient.

Acitretin is a metabolite of etretinate. Acitretin normalizes cell differentiation and thins the cornified layer by directly reducing the keratinocytes' rate of proliferation. It also decreases inflammation in the dermis and epidermis by inhibiting the chemotaxis of polymorphonuclear cells and the release of proinflammatory mediators by neutrophils.[1] In contrast with isotretinoin, acitretin seems to be a promising method for HS management. However, owing to the high daily dosage, its use may be limited.[1] Evidence Category III, Strength of Recommendation C (see **Table 1**).

ALITRETINOIN

Alitretinoin has a similar mode of action as acitretin, but has a shorter half-life. In a case series of 14 patients alitretinoin 10 mg/d for 24 weeks demonstrated a significant improvement in 79% of the cases. Alitretinoin may have a role in the treatment of HS specifically in women of fertile age. Evidence Category IV, Strength of Recommendation D. (see **Table 1**).

RESORCINOL

Topical resorcinol for HS has been studied in 1 prospective case series study.[27] Twelve patients with mild HS were instructed to apply resorcinol 15% twice daily in case of an HS flare. In all patients, the use of resorcinol resulted in a significant decrease in pain as assessed by visual analog scale and reported a reduction in mean duration of the painful abscesses.[27] Topical resorcinol (m-dihydroxy benzene) is an exfoliant that has keratolytic, antipruritic, and antiseptic properties.[27] Topical resorcinol can be useful to shorten the mean duration of a painful nodule or abscess. Evidence Category IV, Strength of Recommendation D (see **Table 1**).

INTRAMUSCULAR GAMMA-GLOBULIN

Intramuscular gamma-globulin injection for HS has been studied in 1 retrospective case series including 5 HS patients.[28] Intramuscular human immunoglobulin was administered at a dose of 12.38 mg/kg for an unknown duration and resulted in a 50% to 70% improvement in 4 of 5 patients.[28] Intramuscular gamma-globulin decreases inflammation by various, mainly antibody-mediated, components of immune mechanisms.[28] Evidence Category IV, Strength of Recommendation D (see **Table 1**).

COLCHICINE

In a small, prospective, pilot study the efficacy of 0.5 mg colchicine twice a day orally was studied in 8 HS patients. The patients were treated up to 4 months.[29] After 1 month, only 2 of 8 patients experienced slight improvement on the Physician Global Assessment, whereas 6 of 8 reported no change. After 2 months, 3 patients slightly improved, 1 worsened, and 2 experienced no change. After 4 months, all but 2 patients dropped out owing to lack of efficacy and adverse side effects. Colchicine inhibits several cytokine signaling pathways. In gout, colchicine suppresses inflammasome-driven caspase-1 activation and IL-1β release. Its efficacy in neutrophilic autoinflammatory diseases is attributed to its effect on neutrophils in addition to the inhibition of the inflammasome.[29] The efficacy of colchicine seems poor and has therefore no place in the treatments of HS. Evidence Category IV, Strength of Recommendation D (see **Table 1**).

METFORMIN

In 2009, a case was published in which an HS patient experienced a flare-up after metformin discontinuation and a subsequent remission after restarting metformin.[30] This case report was followed in 2013 by a case series in which 25 patients with mild HS where treated with metformin over a period of 24 weeks.[31] Eighteen patients significantly reduced their Sartorius score. Metformin was uptitrated from a starting dose of 500 mg once a day in the first week, to 500 mg twice a day in the second week, with a maximum dose of 500 mg 3 times a day introduced from the third week onward. The assumed mode of action of metformin in HS is reducing hyperandrogenism by reducing ovarian overproduction of androgens. Evidence Category III, Strength of Recommendation C (see **Table 1**).

ZINC GLUCONATE

The efficacy of zinc has been studied in one prospective case series in which 22 patients with mild to severe HS were treated with 90 mg of zinc gluconate per day.[32] A clinical response was observed in all patients, with 8 complete remissions and 14 partial remissions. Zinc has demonstrated to induce an alteration of innate immunity in HS skin.[19] Toll-like receptors 2, 3, 4, 7, and 9 intercellular adhesion molecule 1; IL-6, TNF-α, melanocyte-stimulating hormone, transforming growth factor-β, β-defensin 2 and 4, and insulin-like growth factor 1 were all increased toward normal by immunohistochemical analysis after zinc treatment.[33] Evidence Category III, Strength of Recommendation C (see **Table 1**).

BOTULINUM TOXIN

The efficacy of botulinum toxin injections for HS has been reported in 3 case reports.[34–36] In 2 of the 3 cases, positive results were described. The mechanism of how botulinum toxin would ameliorate HS is not known, but it has been speculated that it reduces the moist environment and thus reduces a rich substrate for bacterial growth.[36]

Evidence Category IV, Strength of Recommendation D (see **Table 1**).

TACROLIMUS

Two case reports report on the efficacy of oral tacrolimus in HS.[37,38] In both cases, a patient with a kidney transplantation and comorbid moderate HS received tacrolimus and mycophenolate, and subsequently all HS lesions disappeared.[37,38] This response was attributed to tacrolimus because both patients already used mycophenolate before a switch from cyclosporine to tacrolimus. Its efficacy was attributed to its immune modulating properties. Evidence Category IV, Strength of Recommendation D (see **Table 1**).

FUMARATES

In 1 prospective case series, 7 HS patients with moderate to severe HS were treated with a progressive dosage scheme as a last resort therapy.[39] A meaningful improvement was observed in 3 patients. The mode of action of fumarates in improving HS was thought to be via its immunomodulatory and antiinflammatory effects.[39] Evidence Category IV, Strength of Recommendation D (see **Table 1**).

FUTURE RESEARCH

Many of the treatments discussed have shown initially promising results in case series or case reports and should be studied in more detail using randomized, double-blind, placebo-controlled trials. Preferably the therapy should be compared with proven treatment modality such as oral tetracyclines or an anti–tumor necrosis factor-α therapy that have undergone high-quality assessment and have Category of Evidence of I or II.

We suggest that future studies should include patients who fulfill the Dessau definition, that is, HS is a chronic inflammatory recurrent debilitating skin disease (of the terminal hair follicle) that usually presents after puberty with painful, deep-seated, inflamed lesions in the aplocrine gland-bearing areas of the body most commonly the axillae, inguinal, and anal–genital areas.[1]

Diagnostic criteria such as those presented in the European HS Guidelines should be part of standard inclusion/exclusion criteria.[1] Owing to the fact that a variety of outcome measures have been used over the years, objective, validated outcome measures such as the Hidradenitis Suppurativa Clinical Response, Physician Global Assessment, and other relevant clinical measures should be assessed.[40] In addition to the objective validated clinical scores, validated patient reported outcome measures that include quality of life, pain, and other relevant assessments must be included.[40] Because the severity of HS naturally tends to fluctuate and the disease has a chronic course, primary outcome measures are likely to be based on therapy of 6 or 12 months with long-term follow-up required to assess the therapeutic intervention on the natural history of the disease.

SUMMARY

HS is a common debilitating skin disease that has been neglected by science for many years. Fortunately, the disease is getting more and more attention, which is reflected by the exponentially rising number of scientific publications. Nevertheless, there is a clear need for effective treatment. That being said, we are still at the beginning of improving care for these patients as demonstrated by the low levels of evidence for the medical treatments discussed in this article. Many of these therapies showed promising results, but are still waiting to be validated in randomized, controlled trials. It is clear that much more research is needed to strengthen the Level of Evidence for these therapies and thus improve patient care.

REFERENCES

1. Zouboulis CC, Desai N, Emtestam L, et al. European S1 guideline for the treatment of hidradenitis suppurativa/acne inversa. J Eur Acad Dermatol Venereol 2015;29:619–44.
2. Gulliver WP, Zouboulis CC, Errol Prens EP. Evidence-based approach to the treatment of hidradenitis suppurativa/acne inversa, based on the European Guidelines for Hidradenitis Suppurativa. Reviews of Endocrine and Metabolic Disorders, in press.
3. Gulliver WP, Jemec GB, Baker KA. Experience with ustekinumab for the treatment of moderate to severe hidradenitis suppurativa. J Eur Acad Dermatol Venereol 2012;26(7):911–4.
4. Blok JL, Jonkman MF, Horvath B. Results of the first prospective open label study investigating the effectiveness and safety of usekinumab in hidradenitis suppurativa. EADV Congress. Amsterdam, The Netherlands, October 8–12, 2014.
5. Jemec GBE, Revuz J, Leyden J. Hidradenitis suppurativa. Berlin: Springer; 2006. p. 138–40.
6. Firooz A, Tehranchi-Nia Z, Ahmed AR. Benefits and risks of intralesional corticosteroid injection in the treatment of dermatological diseases. Clin Exp Dermatol 1995;20:363–70.
7. Danto JL. Preliminary studies of the effect of hydrocortisone on hidradenitis suppurativa. J Invest Dermatol 1958;31:299–300.

8. Yazdanyar S, Boer J, Ingvarsson G, et al. Dapsone therapy for hidradenitis suppurativa: a series of 24 patients. Dermatology 2011;222:342–6.
9. Hofer T, Itin PH. Acne inversa: a dapsone-sensitive dermatosis. Hautarzt 2001;52:989–92 [in German].
10. Gupta AK, Ellis CN, Nickoloff BJ, et al. Oral cyclosporine in the treatment of inflammatory and noninflammatory dermatoses. A clinical and immunopathologic analysis. Arch Dermatol 1990;126: 339–50.
11. Rose RF, Goodfield MJ, Clark SM. Treatment of recalcitrant hidradenitis suppurativa with oral ciclosporin. Clin Exp Dermatol 2006;31:154–5.
12. Buckley DA, Rogers S. Cyclosporin-responsive hidradenitis suppurativa. J R Soc Med 1995;88: 289P–90P.
13. Sawers RS, Randall VA, Ebling FJ. Control of hidradenitis suppurativa in women using combined antiandrogen (cyproterone acetate) and oestrogen therapy. Br J Dermatol 1986;115:269–74.
14. Stellon AJ, Wakeling M. Hidradenitis suppurativa associated with use of oral contraceptives. BMJ 1989;298:28–9.
15. Boer J, van Gemert MJ. Long-term results of isotretinoin in the treatment of 68 patients with hidradenitis suppurativa. J Am Acad Dermatol 1999;40:73–6.
16. Soria A, Canoui-Poitrine F, Wolkenstein P, et al. Absence of efficacy of oral isotretinoin in hidradenitis suppurativa: a retrospective study based on patients' outcome assessment. Dermatology 2009; 218:134–5.
17. Fearfield LA, Staughton RC. Severe vulval apocrine acne successfully treated with prednisolone and isotretinoin. Clin Exp Dermatol 1999;24:189–92.
18. Brown CF, Gallup DG, Brown VM. Hidradenitis suppurativa of the anogenital region: response to isotretinoin. Am J Obstet Gynecol 1988;158:12–5.
19. Dicken CH, Powell ST, Spear KL. Evaluation of isotretinoin treatment of hidradenitis suppurativa. J Am Acad Dermatol 1984;11:500–2.
20. Jones DH, Cunliffe WJ, King K. Hidradenitis suppurativa-lack of success with 13-cis-retinoic acid. Br J Dermatol 1982;107:252.
21. Norris JF, Cunliffe WJ. Failure of treatment of familial widespread hidradenitis suppurativa with isotretinoin. Clin Exp Dermatol 1986;11:579–83.
22. Boer J, Nazary M. Long-term results of acitretin therapy for hidradenitis suppurativa. Is acne inversa also a misnomer? Br J Dermatol 2011;164:170–5.
23. Matusiak L, Bieniek A, Szepietowski JC. Acitretin treatment for hidradenitis suppurativa: a prospective series of 17 patients. Br J Dermatol 2014;171:170–4.
24. Hogan DJ, Light MJ. Successful treatment of hidradenitis suppurativa with acitretin. J Am Acad Dermatol 1988;19:355–6.
25. Scheman AJ. Nodulocystic acne and hidradenitis suppurativa treated with acitretin: a case report. Cutis 2002;69:287–8.
26. Chow ET, Mortimer PS. Successful treatment of hidradenitis suppurativa and retroauricular acne with etretinate. Br J Dermatol 1992;126:415.
27. Boer J, Jemec GB. Resorcinol peels as a possible self-treatment of painful nodules in hidradenitis suppurativa. Clin Exp Dermatol 2010;35:36–40.
28. Goo B, Chung HJ, Chung WG, et al. Intramuscular immunoglobulin for recalcitrant suppurative diseases of the skin: a retrospective review of 63 cases. Br J Dermatol 2007;157:563–8.
29. van der Zee HH, Prens EP. The anti-inflammatory drug colchicine lacks efficacy in hidradenitis suppurativa. Dermatology 2011;223:169–73.
30. Arun B, Loffeld A. Long-standing hidradenitis suppurativa treated effectively with metformin. Clin Exp Dermatol 2009;34:920–1.
31. Verdolini R, Clayton N, Smith A, et al. Metformin for the treatment of hidradenitis suppurativa: a little help along the way. J Eur Acad Dermatol Venereol 2013;27:1101–8.
32. Brocard A, Knol AC, Khammari A, et al. Hidradenitis suppurativa and zinc: a new therapeutic approach. A pilot study. Dermatology 2007;214:325–7.
33. Dreno B, Khammari A, Brocard A, et al. Hidradenitis suppurativa: the role of deficient cutaneous innate immunity. Arch Dermatol 2012;148:182–6.
34. O'Reilly DJ, Pleat JM, Richards AM. Treatment of hidradenitis suppurativa with botulinum toxin A. Plast Reconstr Surg 2005;116:1575–6.
35. Feito-Rodriguez M, Sendagorta-Cudos E, Herranz-Pinto P, et al. Prepubertal hidradenitis suppurativa successfully treated with botulinum toxin A. Dermatol Surg 2009;35:1300–2.
36. Khoo AB, Burova EP. Hidradenitis suppurativa treated with *Clostridium botulinum* toxin A. Clin Exp Dermatol 2014;39:749–50.
37. Ducroux E, Ocampo MA, Kanitakis J, et al. Hidradenitis suppurativa after renal transplantation: complete remission after switching from oral cyclosporine to oral tacrolimus. J Am Acad Dermatol 2014;71:e210–1.
38. Arnadottir M, Jonsson E, Jonsson J. Inactivity of hidradenitis suppurativa after renal transplantation. Transplantation 2006;82:849.
39. Deckers IE, van der Zee HH, Balak DM, et al. Fumarates, a new treatment option for therapy-resistant hidradenitis suppurativa: a prospective open-label pilot study. Br J Dermatol 2015;172:828–9.
40. Kimball AB, Jemec GEB, Yang M, et al. Assessing the validity, responsiveness and meaningfulness of the Hidradenitis Suppurativa Clinical Response (HiSCR) as the clinical endpoint for hidradenitis suppurativa treatment. Br J Dermatol 2014;171:1434–42.

Surgical Procedures in Hidradenitis Suppurativa

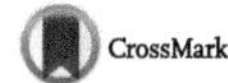

Ineke Janse, MD[a,*], Andrzej Bieniek, MD, PhD[b], Barbara Horváth, MD, PhD[a], Łukasz Matusiak, MD, PhD[b]

KEYWORDS

• Deroofing • STEEP • Wide excision • Closure techniques • Surgery • Hidradenitis suppurativa

KEY POINTS

- At least in higher stages of hidradenitis suppurativa (HS), surgery should be introduced early after setting the diagnosis.
- Preoperatively, immunosuppressive and/or antibacterial medical treatment to calm active inflammation must be considered. Imaging (ultrasonography, MRI) may be helpful.
- Depending on the extent and severity of the disease local, tumescent, spinal, and/or general anesthesia are used.
- Acute phase surgical treatment and treatment of the chronic continue intermediary phase should be distinguished. Incision and drainage can offer pain relief from a tense fluctuating acute abscess.
- After wide excision, different wound closure techniques can be chosen. Secondary intention healing usually ensures good functional/cosmetic results in defects up to 140 cm^2.
- Deroofing, 'skin-tissue-saving excision with electrosurgical peeling' (STEEP) and wide excision are preferred surgical methods for the chronic phase.

INTRODUCTION

Hidradenitis suppurativa (HS) is difficult to treat owing to its complex pathomechanism; beside the extensive inflammation with abscesses and inflammatory nodules, there is also sinus tract formation and in severe cases extensive scarring.[1] Surgery should be introduced early in the management of HS. Unfortunately, surgical treatment is often performed many years after the initial symptoms of the disease, after numerous ineffective cycles of pharmacotherapy.[2] Such delays are often caused by misdiagnosis, a doctor's lack of knowledge about the disease, unjustified confidence in the efficacy of noninvasive therapies, anxiety about surgical treatment and the embarrassing location.[3] The tolerance to and satisfaction with, sometimes debilitating, surgical procedures is surprisingly high and may result from the large psychosocial impact of HS. Because the magnitude of life impairment in HS is far greater than in other dermatoses, patients are highly willing to change the condition.[4,5]

TREATMENT GOALS AND PLANNED OUTCOMES

The comparison of different operative methods of HS is difficult because of the many types of surgery, interindividual differences between patients and between operators, the shortage of randomized trials, and the lack of consensus about the endpoints used. To be able to compare different surgical interventions, clear definitions of outcomes should be defined. We therefore suggest outcomes for future studies.

Disclosures: Dr B. Horváth performed investigator initiative studies of Jansen Cilag B.V. (The Netherlands) and Abbvie Inc. Further, she received unrestricted educational grant from Abbvie Netherlands (The Netherlands).
[a] Department of Dermatology, University Medical Center Groningen, University of Groningen, Hanzeplein 1, Groningen 9700 RB, The Netherlands; [b] Department of Dermatology, Wroclaw Medical University, University of Wrocław, Chalubinskiego 1, 50-368 Wrocław, Poland
* Corresponding author.
E-mail address: i.c.janse@umcg.nl

Dermatol Clin 34 (2016) 97–109
http://dx.doi.org/10.1016/j.det.2015.08.007
0733-8635/16/$ – see front matter

Relapse Rates

Relapse (owing to nonradical surgery) is defined as inflammatory activity occurring within 0.5 cm of the surgical scar. The natural progression of HS can be defined as inflammation that develops outside this area but in the same anatomic region.[6]

Time to Wound Closure

The time to wound closure is defined as the duration of the wound healing (complete healing) measured in days. For sutured lesions, complete healing may be considered achieved when stitches have been removed.

Complications

Early complications include hemorrhage, infection, hypergranulation, necrosis of grafts or flaps, injury of brachial plexus or big axillary vessels, and thrombosis of brachial veins.[2] Late complications include wound dehiscence, retention of serum (seroma), cicatricial contracture, hypertrophic scars, and keloids.[2,3,7]

Patient-Reported Outcomes

Patient satisfaction can be cosmetic or functional. The rate of either is measured on a numerical rating scale of 1 to 10, where 1 corresponds with very dissatisfied and 10 with excellent. If the satisfaction rate is measured for both functional and cosmetic results, the mean rate is shown. The recommendation of the treatment to other people and willingness to undergo further surgery are also important patient-reported outcomes.

PREOPERATIVE PLANNING AND PREPARATION

Medication to Calm the Inflammation

In moderate and severe HS, it is broadly recommended and accepted that surgery is combined with immunomodulating treatment. However, it remains unclear whether relapse rates after surgery with perioperative immunomodulation therapy are lower than surgical treatments without perioperative medication.[8]

Imaging

Imaging is not used routinely in surgery for HS, although it may be beneficial to management.[9] Some studies with ultrasonography showed that the inflammation can be extended horizontally and vertically far over the visible borders of the inflammation on the skin surface.[10] Moreover, differentiating between enterocutaneous fistula formation in Crohn's disease remains challenging, especially in the perianal region. Perianal lesions of Crohn's disease usually present as wide fistulas, entering deeply through the perianal area to the colon and/or vagina, affecting the skin and subcutaneous tissue only to a small extent. Lesions of HS present as purulent, inflammatory infiltrates, frequently reaching the buttocks and perineum with numerous narrow, less visible shallow fistulas reaching the anus. Moreover, mixed clinical presentations can occur because of coexistence of HS and Crohn's disease.[11]

In ambiguous cases, imaging with ultrasonography, MRI, CT, and fistulography are helpful to assess the location and depth of fistulas and sinuses. Shallow lesions expressing the features of HS can be treated surgically by a (dermato)surgeon, independent from the established diagnosis of Crohn's disease. If the diagnosis of Crohn's disease with deep fistulas is confirmed, the surgical treatment should be carried out in cooperation with proctologic specialists. The diagnostic imaging, primarily fistulography, may be decisive.

PATIENT POSITIONING

Surgery involving the axillae and mons pubis is performed in supine position. Leg rests are used for operating inguinal and perineal lesions. The patient is placed in prone position during operations on perianal and gluteal HS.

PROCEDURAL APPROACH

Anesthesia

Local anesthesia

Local anesthesia is performed in 2 steps. First, field block anesthesia is performed with lidocaine 1% (10 mg/mL) plus adrenaline (5 μg/mL). Second, nodules and/or sinus tracts are injected with the same local anesthetic. If patients have a fear of needles or if they experience a lot of pain during local anesthesia, lidocaine and prilocaine cream (eutectic mixture of local anesthetics [EMLA]) can be applied 1 hour before the injections.[6]

Tumescent local anesthesia

In tumescent local anesthesia (TLA), large volumes (≥100 mL) of highly diluted local anesthetics (usually lidocaine buffered with sodium bicarbonate) are injected subdermally with mechanical assistance.[12] In simple cases, it may be used as the sole method of anesthesia; in more advanced cases, it can be combined with sedation, spinal, or general anesthesia. Because of the necessity of large skin incisions and difficulty in diffusion in indurated, fibrotic tissue, the concentration of lidocaine should be relatively high (0.1%), especially when TLA is used as the sole form of anesthesia.

If TLA is used as a complementary agent, the concentration of lidocaine may be as low as 0.04% to 0.05%. Because the absorption of lidocaine is expected to be relatively high in lesional HS tissue, a maximal dose of 35 mg/kg lidocaine is recommended.[13] The concentration of other components of TLA solution are as usual: adrenaline (1:1–2 million) and sodium bicarbonate (10–20 mL in 1000 mL 0.9% NaCl). The tumescent solution is injected abundantly with use of a rotation pump, special tubing, and long (spinal) needles. Owing to specific properties of TLA, intraoperative and postoperative bleeding is greatly reduced, ensuring accurate and safe surgery and minimal blood loss, and the risk of infection is diminished owing to antiseptic activity of bicarbonate and the wash away of infectious agents by copious discharge of fluid from the wound. Finally, postoperative pain is decreased for many hours (**Fig. 1**).[14]

General and spinal anesthesia

Under general and spinal anesthesia, large areas can be operated on without the limitation of the maximum allowed amount of local anesthetics. In addition, some patients favor general anesthesia above local anesthesia, which can be painful and difficult to achieve in areas of active inflammation and fibrosis.

Lesion Removal Techniques

Incision and drainage

The purpose of incision and drainage is pain relief in case of a tense, fluctuating acute abscess. There is only a short-term effect, because lesions treated by incision and drainage tend to relapse.[15] For drainage, 6- to 8-mm punch biopsies can be used. By digital pressure and rinsing with saline solution, the remaining pus is removed.

Deroofing

The deroofing technique was first described by Mullins and colleagues[16] in 1959. In the 1980s, the technique was modified by preservation of the exposed lesion floor.[17,18] Presently, there is a tendency to remove keratinous debris and viable epithelial remnants on the floor because these substances could cause relapses when left present. Deroofing is the primary surgical therapy for persisting nodules or sinus tracts in HS Hurley stage I/II.[6] The procedure starts with identification of the HS lesions to be deroofed by physical examination. Local anesthesia is performed as described under Medication to Calm the Inflammation and Imaging. Next, a blunt probe is used to identify sinus openings. After introduction, the probe is placed at different angels in search of connecting fistulas. The probe should be inserted into the fistula without resistance. If force is applied, false tracts can be created with the probe. The sinus roof is removed using electrosurgical dissection with a wire loop tip coupled to an electrosurgical generator (**Fig. 2**). The probe is used as a guide, leaving the epithelial bottom of the sinus tract intact. The margins must be probed again for residual communicating sinus tracts. The jelly-like material on the floor of the sinus tract needs to be removed superficially with the wire loop tip. The defects are left open for healing by secondary intention.[6,19]

Skin-tissue–saving excision with electrosurgical peeling

This surgical technique for HS was described by Blok and colleagues[20]: the skin-tissue–saving excision with electrosurgical peeling (STEEP) procedure. STEEP seems to be a promising alternative to wide excision in extensive disease because it saves healthy tissue to a maximum

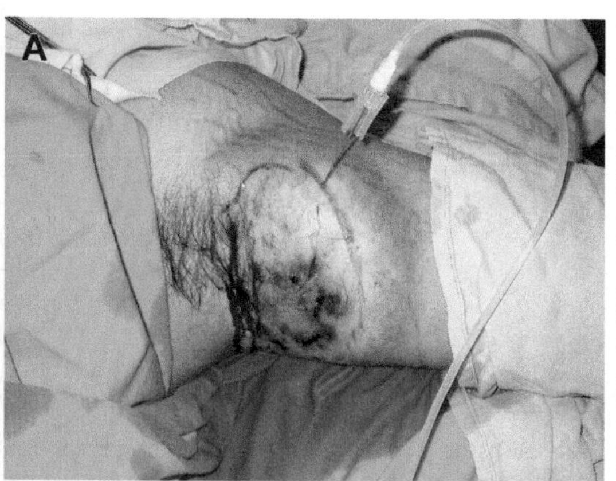

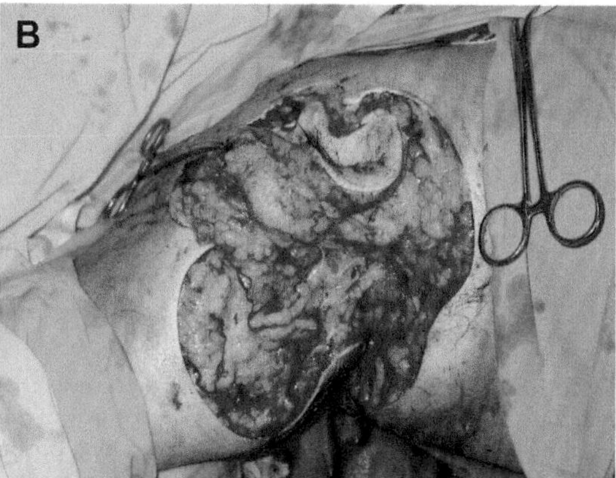

Fig. 1. (*A*) Infiltration of the axilla with tumescent local anesthesia. (*B*) Tumescent local anesthesia reduces bleeding and enhances visualization.

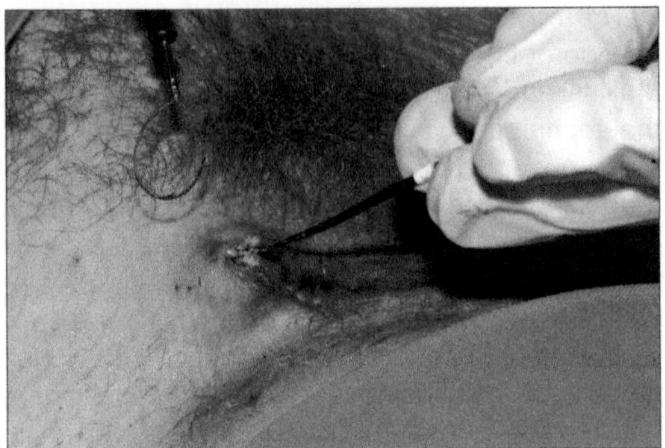

Fig. 2. Sinus roof is removing by electrosurgical dissection in the deroofing procedure.

and achieves complete removal of lesional tissue (**Fig. 3**).[20] The idea is that tissue sparing leads to quick wound healing, good cosmetic results, and low risk of contractures. Recurrence rates seem similar to wide excision because both techniques are aimed at complete removal of lesional and fibrotic tissue.[8,20] STEEP is performed mostly under general anesthesia. Preoperatively, the operation field is palpated and sinus tracts are probed to get an impression about the extent of the disease. Next, the sinus roofs are incised electrosurgically with a wire loop tip coupled to an electrosurgical generator. Subsequently, successive tangential excisions are made until the epithelialized floor of the sinus tract is reached. Tangential peeling off affected tissue is continued until the area is clear of lesional tissue and fibrosis. Thereafter, the wound edges are checked with a probe for remaining sinus tracts. During and after the procedure, hemostasis is achieved by using the coagulation mode of the Erbotoom. Finally, the margins of the wound can be injected with triamcinolonacetonide 10 to 20 mg to prevent hypergranulation and bupivacaine 0.5% (10 mL) for postoperative analgesia. The defects are left open for healing by secondary intention (**Fig. 4**).

Excision

Excision is aimed at complete removal of lesions. The extent of pathologic lesions should be determined by observation in bright illumination and palpation showing the leakage of pus after compression. Furthermore symptoms reported by the patient should be taken into consideration, like localized pain and drainage.

Different surgical approaches are used with varying degrees of invasiveness. In limited local excision, each separate lesion is excised with a certain margin of healthy tissue. In wide excision, an area embracing all lesions is removed. In radical excision, an entire area of a body region in which the disease may presumable spread is excised.[21] For all 3 techniques, often a lateral margin of 1 cm is proposed.[2] However, in small lesions, to ensure complete removal, a sparse margin may be sufficient. There is no consensus about whether partial or complete removal of the subcutaneous fat should be achieved.[2] It is advised to adjust the excision to the extent and severity of the disease, as well as to the dynamics of its development. Particularly at depth, in proximity of big neurovascular bundles in axillary and inguinal regions, as well as around the rectum, overzealous excisions should be avoided. The complications of such interventions may cause more morbidity than the disease itself (**Fig. 5**). That is why recommendation for curettage of any remaining walls of sinuses is given, instead of thorough excision in these cases (**Fig. 6**).

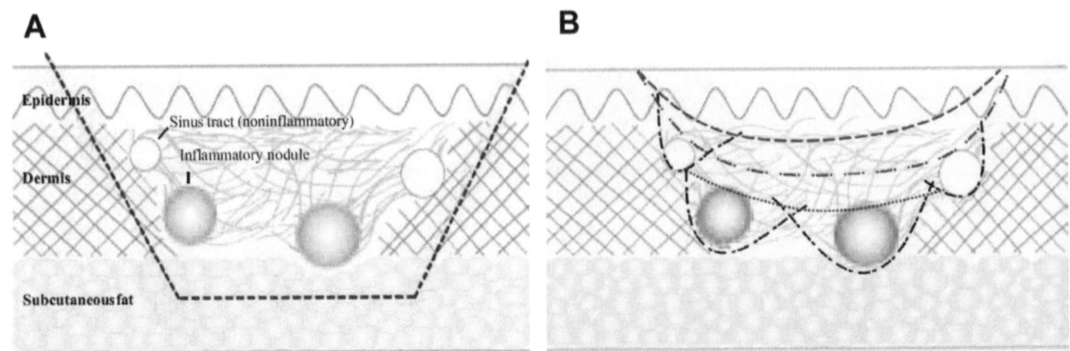

Fig. 3. (*A*) Wide excision: red dotted line represents the cutting plane. Healthy skin and subcutis are removed. (*B*) The skin-tissue–sparing excision with electrosurgical peeling (STEEP) procedure: nodules and scar tissue are identified by palpation, sinus tracts are localized by a probe. Diseased tissue is removed by means of tangential transections (*red dashed lines*). The defect is smaller compared with wide excision. (*From* Blok JL, Spoo JR, Leeman FW, et al. Skin-tissue-sparing excision with electrosurgical peeling (STEEP): A surgical treatment option for severe hidradenitis suppurativa Hurley stage II/III. Eur Acad Dermatol Venereol 2015;29(2):380; with permission.)

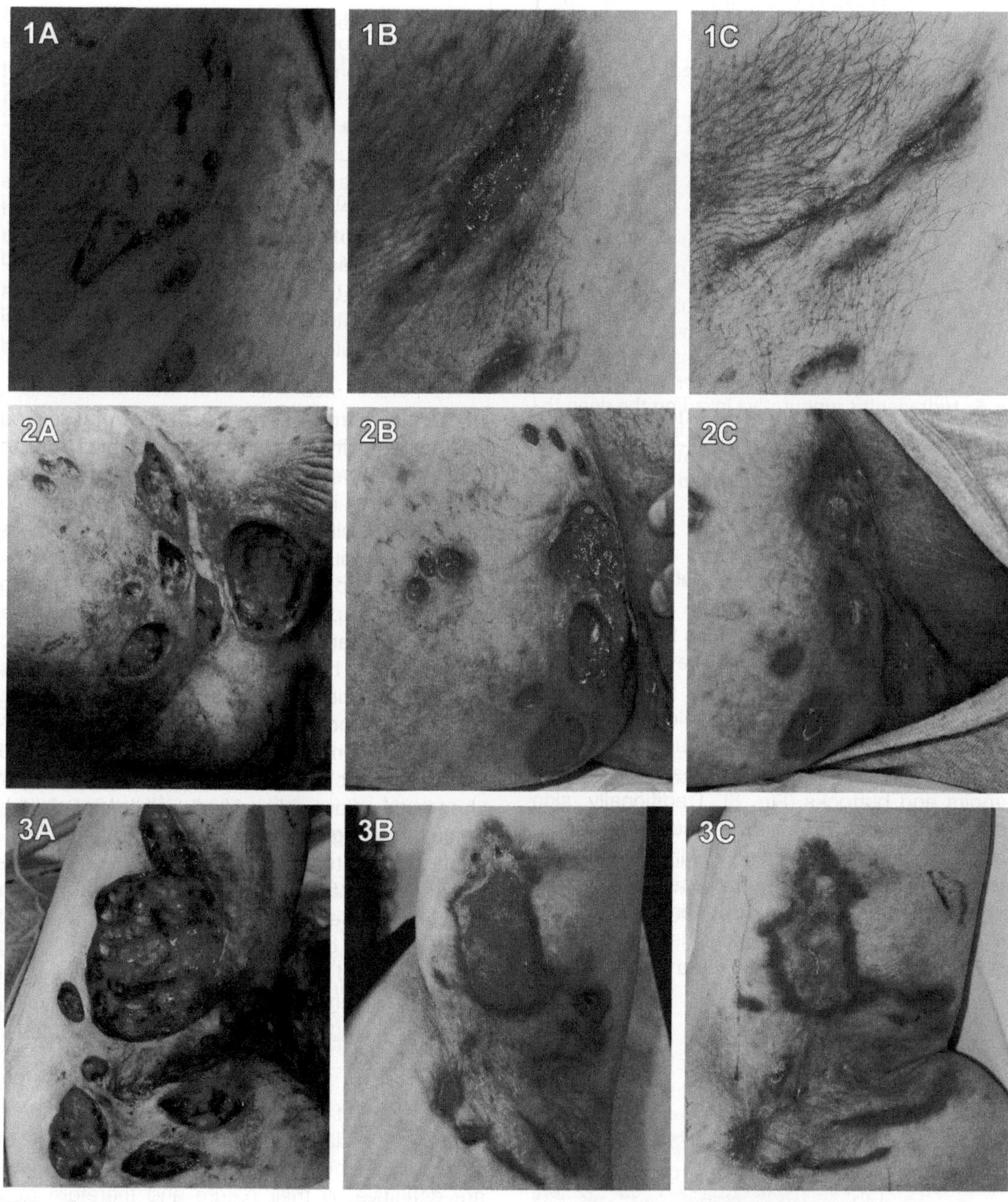

Fig. 4. Cosmetic result of skin-tissue–sparing excision with electrosurgical peeling (STEEP). (*1A–C*) Axilla of a 47-year-old man, Hurley stage II. (*2A–C*) Groin of a 46-year-old man, Hurley stage II. (*3A–C*) Axilla of a 49-year-old woman, Hurley stage III.

Wound Closure Techniques

Primary closure

Sutures Simple sutures may be recommended in small defects surrounded by loose skin. Undermining as well as suturing under high tension should be avoided, because of risk of healing disturbances. This option usually ensures fast healing with good cosmetic and functional results (**Fig. 7**).[22] It is advisable to close the wound rather loosely, which enables the outflow of exudate and limits risk of infection.

Split-thickness skin grafts Split-thickness skin grafts, usually meshed, are used typically in large wounds.[23,24] Grafts of 0.6 to 0.8 mm thickness

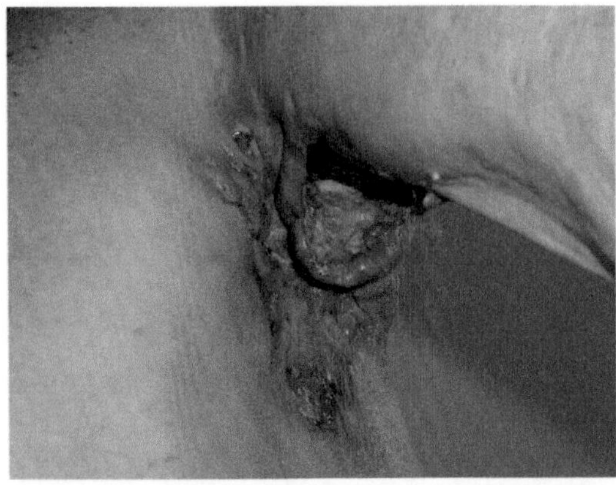

Fig. 5. Hidradenitis suppurativa invading the deep tissues of the axillary area. During excision, the weakened axillary artery was accidentally damaged, which required further suturing and coverage with skin-fascial flap.

are harvested from the thighs or buttocks with use of dermatomes, and then they are expanded in a ratio of 3:1 by multiple incisions in the mesh graft device. Grafts allow for closure of even the largest wounds with minimal risk of serious complications. Despite evident differences of color and texture with surrounding skin, they ensure acceptable functional and aesthetic results, especially in the armpits and buttocks (**Fig. 8**). Traditionally, skin grafts were put on granulation tissue, after longer period of wound conditioning. Owing to good hemostatic properties, TLA grafting can also be performed in 1 procedure, directly after excision. Only on genital and inguinal regions is skin grafting made on previously granulated wound bed because of the high risk of infection. Morgan and colleagues[25] compared split skin grafting and secondary intention healing (SIH) in 10 patients undergoing bilateral excision for axillary HS. In each patient, 1 axilla was grafted and the other was allowed for SIH using a Silastic foam dressing. Split skin grafting had a shorter time to wound closure than SIH. However, a majority of patients preferred SIH because of the comfort during healing, limb freedom, and lack of a painful donor site. Additionally, SIH leads to good cosmetic results, whereas skin grafting often gives a patchwork appearance with a persistent depression at the site of excision.[26]

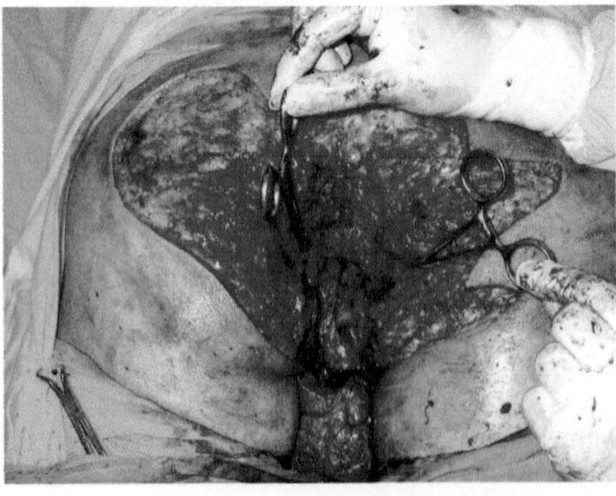

Fig. 6. Deep sinuses entering the perirectal space, accompanying advanced infiltrations of hidradenitis suppurativa located on buttocks. These were opened and curetted, instead of thorough excision. This led to good healing, with no persistent discharge or fistulas.

Flaps Reconstruction with use of flaps may ensure the best quality of skin, owing to thick tissue coverage. Nevertheless, in larger wounds, flaps are difficult or impossible to use. In comparison with grafts, their harvesting is more difficult, more invasive, and subject to risk of serious complications like flap necrosis and hemorrhage. In contrast, this approach is mandatory for coverage of important anatomic structures, like exposed neurovascular bundles. The many forms of flaps that are described in the treatment of HS by a number of authors are shown in **Table 1**. The genital area in women is specifically suitable for the use of flap techniques. The use of pubic–lower abdominal flaps (modified abdominoplasty), obtained during the procedure similar to abdominoplasty, results in accelerated healing and minimized deformations of the vulva and groin (**Fig. 9**).[27,28] Because of the risk of ischemia of distant portion of those flaps, careful undermining and thinning of the tissues is advised. In inguinal areas the thigh advancement flaps, resembling the medial thigh lift technique are successfully used (**Fig. 10**).[29] In axillary areas, they were used exclusively for coverage of exposed big vessels (in the form of fasciocutaneous random pattern transposition flaps). Apart from that, the use of flaps in HS operations should be limited. Flaps are definitive by their nature and therefore may be not appropriate to this medical condition with significant risk of progression. In addition, in HS there is often an underestimation of the defect size preoperatively. Therefore, the proposed flap can be too small.

Healing by secondary intention

SIH may be successful in defects up to 140 cm^2 (Janse and colleagues, unpublished data, 2015; see **Fig. 4**; **Fig. 11**). SIH occurs along with the natural processes of granulation, wound shrinkage, and epithelization. This approach is typically used in the anogenital region, trunk, and axillary

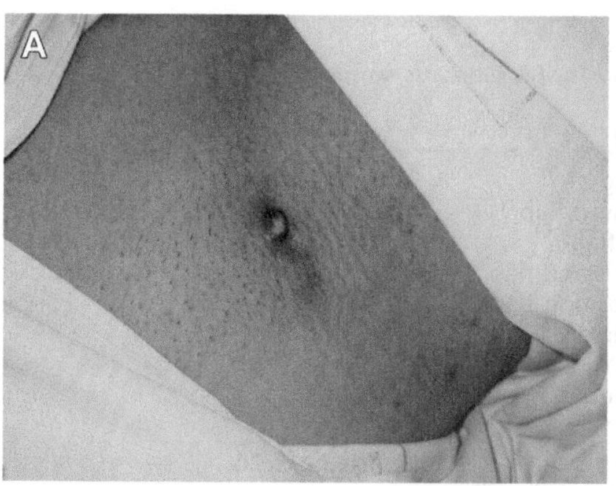

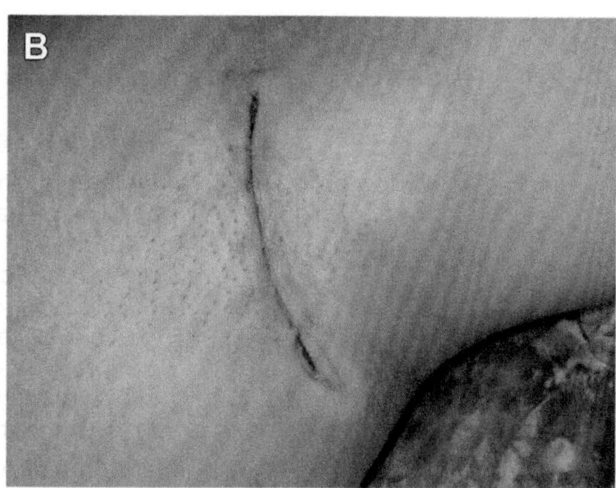

Fig. 7. (*A*) Small abscesses and fistulas of the axillary area, planned for spindle-shaped excision. (*B*) The defect after spindle excision was sutured loosely with subepidermal stitches.

area.[28] SIH ensures usually good functional and cosmetic results (see **Figs. 4** and **11**). Moreover, the final scar has considerably smaller dimensions in comparison with the initial defect.[25] This approach is usually well-tolerated by patients owing to the minimal number of wounds (absence of donor sites) and amazingly unproblematic course of healing (except for the first difficult days).[25,28,42] Its major drawbacks are long healing duration (mean, 6–12 weeks), the risk of unsightly scars in extensive defects, and the development of contractures over flexion areas. Of note, the most important factor responsible for healing period is the size of the wound. The localization was not relevant.[43,44]

Combined reconstructions

By using different techniques simultaneously, the benefits of the individual techniques can be combined. For example, wounds can be partially sutured while leaving its remaining portion for secondary healing. Such an approach was used many times in a closure technique called the starlike technique: the pathologic areas of axillary area are excised, 5 equilateral triangles adjacent to the defect are cut off and resulting defects are sutured (**Fig. 12**). The wound area is hereby diminished by 50% to 80% and resulting in accelerated healing assessed as 6 to 8 weeks.[28] Sutures in combination with skin grafting or partial flap reconstructions with SIH can also give good results.

COMPLICATIONS AFTER SURGERY

Brachial plexus damage and thrombosis are the earliest complications, occurring instantly. Surgical repair of brachial plexus nerves should take place within 3 to 6 months after the injury. The treatment of thrombosis of brachial veins comprises anticoagulant therapy and compression. In case of hemorrhage, another early complication, pressure should be applied to the wound should for 30 minutes. If bleeding continues after 30 minutes, the hemorrhage site must be located. Small bleeders can be coagulated, whereas large vessels require legation. If a wound infection occurs, usually after a few days, a choice should be made between prescribing local or systemic antibiotics.

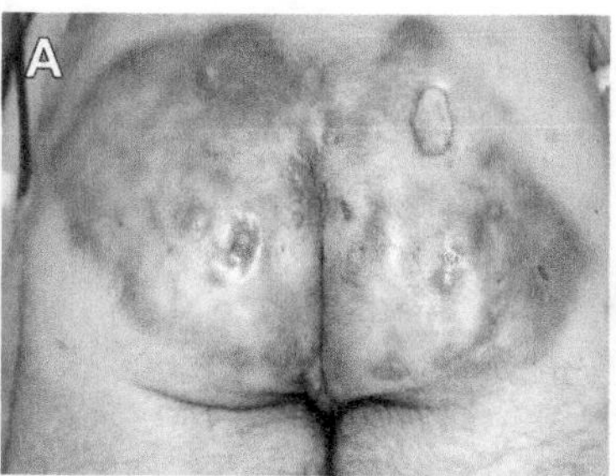

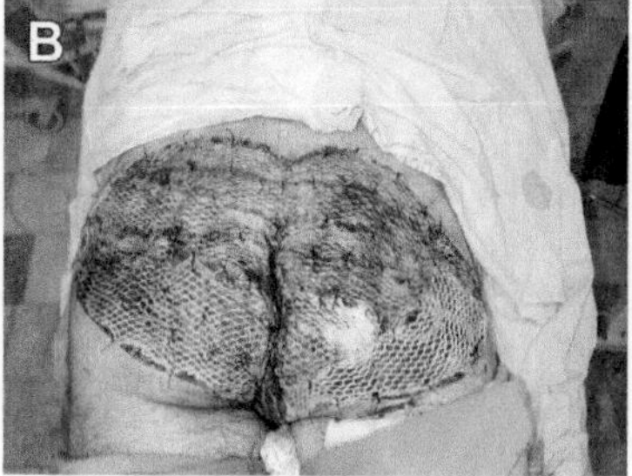

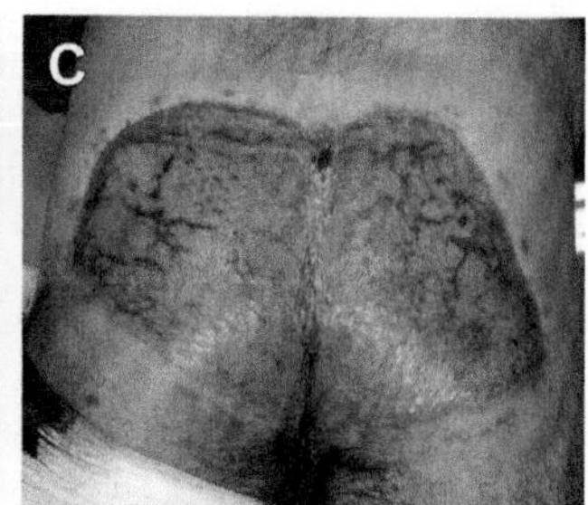

Fig. 8. (*A*) Wide infiltrations of HS in gluteal areas, planned for surgical treatment. (*B*) Directly after excision of the pathologic lesions, wound was covered by meshed split-thickness skin grafts. (*C*) The acceptable scars 1.5 months after the operation (the red-bluish color subsided later).

Table 1
Overview of different types of flaps used in surgery for hidradenitis suppurativa

	Lipocutaneous	Fasciocutaneous	Musculocutaneous	Free
Axillary	Transposition flap of Limberg[30]	Double opposing V–Y perforated based flap[31] Transpositional flap[32] Lateral thoracic island flap[33] Limberg transposition flap[34] Thoracodorsal artery perforator V–Y musculocutaneous advancement flap[35]	Latissimus dorsi island flap[36]	Anterolateral thigh perforator free flap[37]
Groin, perineal, perianal	Modified abdominoplasty[27] Medial thigh lift[29]	Bilateral pedicled anterolateral thigh flap[38]	Pedicled gracilis myocutaneous flap[39]	—
Gluteal	—	Island V–Y advancement flap, rotation V–Y advancement flap and bilobed flap[40] Superior and inferior gluteal artery perforator flaps[41]	—	—

Late complications can also occur. In major dehiscence, the wounds require resuturing. However, most dehiscence can be treated conservatively by allowing the wound to heal by granulation and contraction. Here, it is important to ensure the prevention of infections. Small seromas do not require therapy, whereas large collections should be drained. Debridement may be necessary for necrosis of grafts or flaps. Hypergranulation can be treated with a potent steroid twice daily for 5 days or just can be removed by curettage. Triamcinolonacetonide 10 mg/mL can be injected 3 to 5 times with intervals of 4 weeks in hypertrophic scars or keloid. Serious therapeutic problems may arise from the presence of severe contractures, accompanying axillary HS. In such interventions, despite the usual excision of affected tissue, it is necessary to release the cicatricial contractures (**Fig. 13**). This release is usually done by transection of fibrotic strands adjacent to walls of fistulas and sinuses, with concomitant redression of the shoulder joint. If contracture persists for a long time, the complete correction is very difficult. The contractures can also be corrected using a Z-plasty or skin grafts. The comorbidities and complications of HS are discussed by Miller and colleagues.[43]

POSTPROCEDURAL CARE

In deroofing and STEEP, postoperative care consists of twice daily irrigation followed by alginate

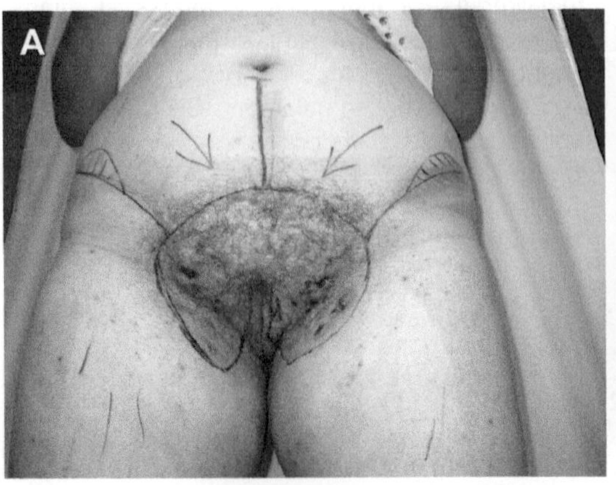

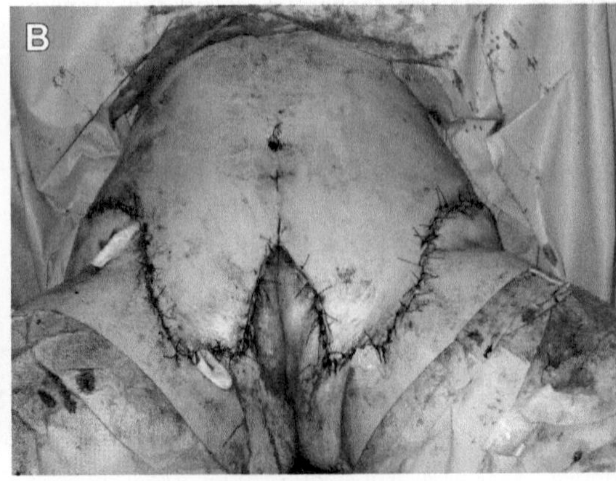

Fig. 9. (*A*) Hidradenitis suppurativa of the genital regions (pubic mound, labia majora, inguinal regions), planned for excision and subsequent coverage with "pubic–lower abdominal" flaps. (*B*) The defect directly after coverage with lower abdominal advancement flaps.

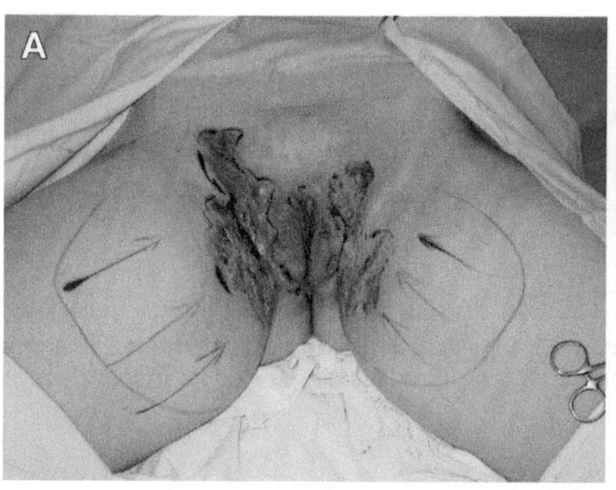

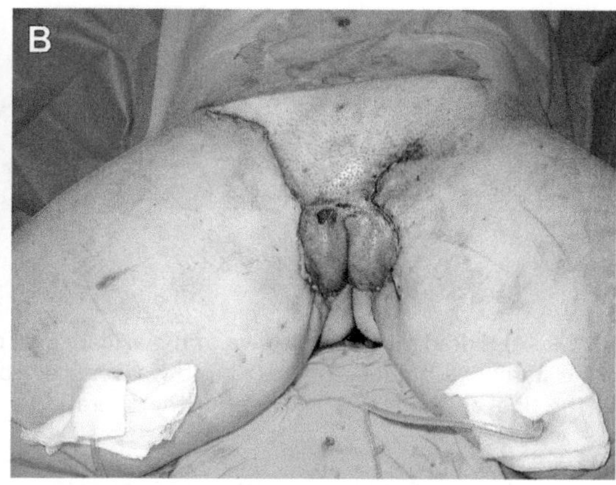

Fig. 10. (*A*) Hidradenitis suppurativa of the genital regions (inguinal and labia majora), planned for excision and coverage with medial thigh lift flaps. (*B*) The defect was covered with skin–subcutaneous medial thigh advancement flaps.

and silicone dressings.[6,20] The large wounds left for SIH could be covered using thick absorbing dressings made of gauze soaked in mixture of petroleum jelly and liquid paraffin (1:1). They are usually removed after 48 to 72 hours and then replaced every 2 days during the first week and later on once a day. In the first week, wounds are managed in sterile conditions—rinsed with use of water disinfecting solution (eg, povidone iodine, boric acid, octenidine). In the following weeks, wounds should be carefully washed with tap water and disinfectant liquid soap, rinsed with octenidine or 3% hydrogen peroxide, dried, smeared with petroleum jelly, and covered with absorbing gauze. Oral antibiotics should be not administered routinely. In the first postoperative week, it is usually necessary to administer oral pain medications to HS sufferers.[43]

After skin grafting, negative pressure dressings can be used. These dressing can increase oxygen levels in the wound, decrease the growth of bacteria, improve granulation, and keep the graft in place in curved areas. A 95% of graft take was seen after using negative pressure dressings.[45,46]

REHABILITATION AND RECOVERY

In many cases, multistaged, prolonged surgical treatment is needed. That is why optimal therapy requires the participation of family physician and public health nurses, as well as assistance and acceptance from the family. Lifestyle measures include losing weight in case of obesity and discontinuing smoking. To prevent cicatricial contractures, it is advisable to introduce physical therapy and physiotherapy subsequent to surgery. Depending on the size of the operation, the time until full recovery to preoperative activity ranges between 4 (Janse and colleagues, unpublished data, 2015) and 10 weeks.[47]

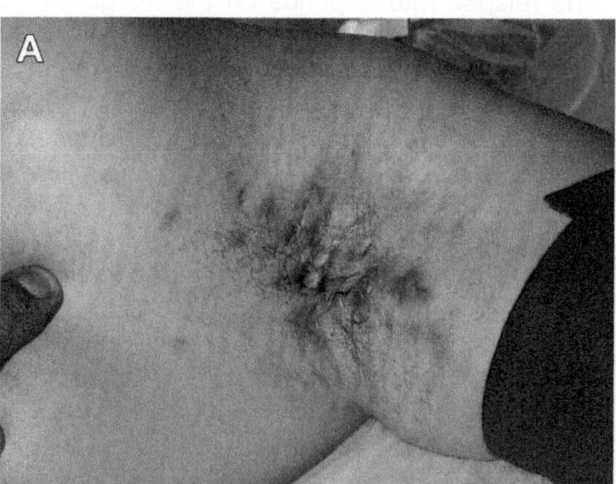

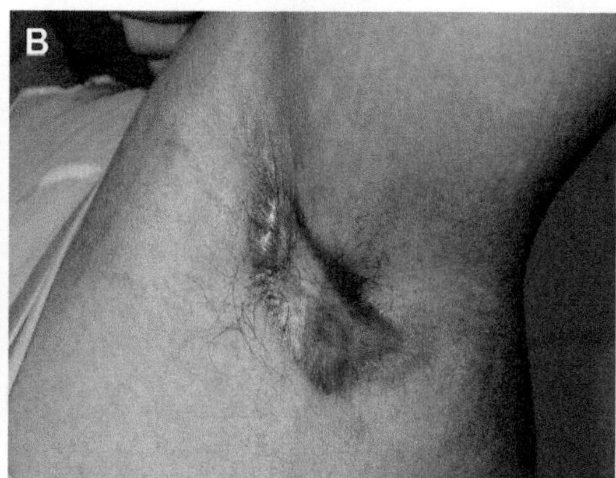

Fig. 11. (*A*) Hidradenitis suppurativa of axillary area, planned for surgical treatment. (*B*) The scar 3 months after completing secondary intention healing. Its size is much smaller than the primary defect.

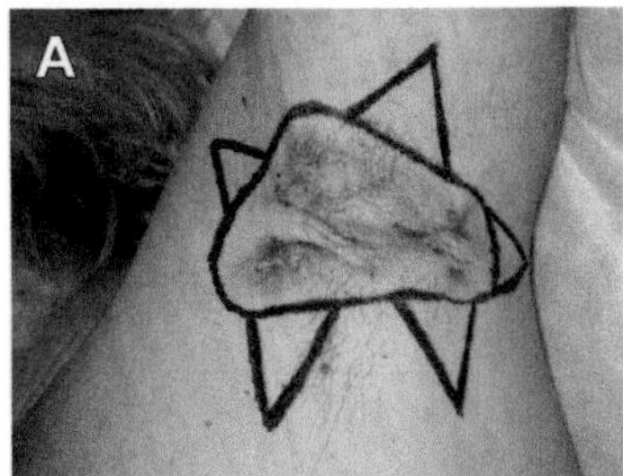

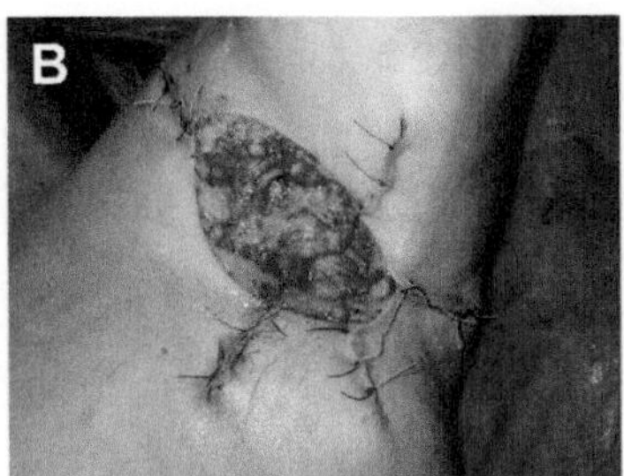

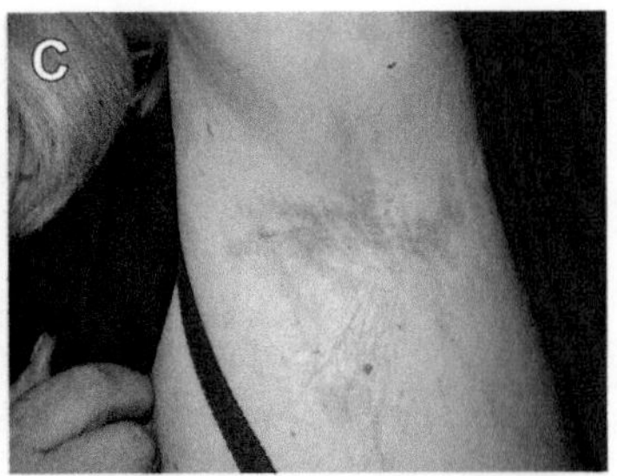

Fig. 12. (*A*) Hidradenitis suppurativa of the axillary area planned for excision with 5 adjacent triangles, according to the starlike technique. (*B*) The wound was reduced considerably by approximating the edges of the triangles. (*C*) The final aesthetic scar 1 year after the operation.

OUTCOMES AND CLINICAL RESULTS IN THE LITERATURE

The results of important outcomes of deroofing, STEEP, and excision are summarized in **Table 2**.

Deroofing

From 2003 to 2007, van der Zee and colleagues[6] treated 44 Hurley I and II HS patients with the deroofing technique. The mean time to wound closure was 14 days at a mean defect length of 3 cm. Of the 88 operated locations, 15 (17%) experienced a relapse after a median of 4.6 months. A lower relapse rate of 4% during a follow-up period of 10 years was reported by Boer and colleagues[48] van der Zee and colleagues[6] described 1 complication in the form of postoperative bleeding; no infections or impairment of movement caused by postoperative scarring were seen. The median satisfaction rate was 8, and 90% of the patients would recommend the technique to other patients.

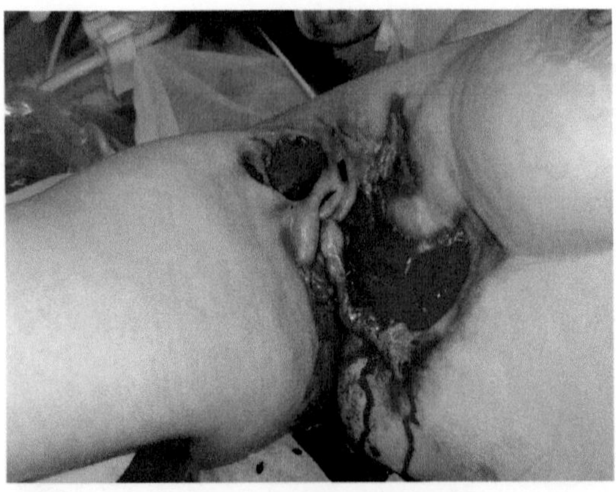

Fig. 13. Chronic hidradenitis suppurativa in axillary location causing significant contracture. The hardened, fibrotic strands must be transected, and contracture released.

Skin-tissue–Saving Excision With Electrosurgical Peeling

In a prospective case series (Janse and colleagues, unpublished data, 2015), the mean time to complete wound healing was 53 days with a median defect size of 15 cm^2. The size of the wound and the Hurley stage were independent predictors for wound healing. A retrospective analysis on 363 deroofings and STEEPs under general anesthesia showed 34% natural progression and 29% relapses owing to irradical surgery.[8] The relapse rate was much lower in the prospective case series in which only 1 of the 27 operation sites relapsed. Hypergranulation is the most common complication. The hypergranulation is usually mild with good reaction to topical treatment with superpotent topical steroids. Wound infections, nerve irritation, postoperative bleeding, and stricture formation are seen very rarely.[8] With a functional outcome of 8.7, a cosmetic outcome of 7.2% and 100% of the patients that would recommend STEEP to others, patients are generally satisfied with the STEEP procedure (see **Fig. 4**).

Excision

The relapse rate depends on the margin of the excision. After limited excision, the relapse rate is 42.8% with a disease-free interval of 11 months. Wide excision has a relapse of 27% after 20 months.[49] The time to wound closure after excision is 6.6 weeks (range, 2–12) with a mean size of the wounds of 40.6 cm^2.[42] Bieniek and colleagues[28] performed 229 operations among 182 patients. During the 1-year follow-up period, complete recovery was observed in 60% of the patients; 31.5% had new but less severe lesions in an adjacent area or at the site of the surgical intervention and 8.5% of the patients showed no improvement. The nature and frequency of complications were similar to those described by others with 7% postoperative bleeding, 10.9% infections, 7% contractures, 32.7% excessive pain,

Table 2
Overview of outcomes of different type of techniques used in surgery for hidradenitis suppurativa

	Deroofing	STEEP	Excision
Indication	Hurley I/II	Hurley II/III	Hurley II/III
Relapse (%)[a]	4–17	3.7–29	27–42.8
Patient reported outcomes[b]			
Satisfaction rate	8	8	—
Recommendation of the treatment to other people (%)	90	100	89.5
Willingness to undergo further surgery (%)	—	—	84
Complications[a]	Postoperative bleeding (1.1%)	Hypergranulation (mild; 62.4%) Postoperative bleeding (1.9%), infections (1.9%), contractures (0.6%), excessive pain (1%), nerve irritation (1%)	Postoperative bleeding (7%), infections (10.9%), contractures (7%), excessive pain (32.7%), wound dehiscence (3.5%)

Abbreviation: STEEP, skin-tissue–sparing excision with electrosurgical peeling.
[a] Percent of total operations.
[b] Percent of patients.

and 3.5% wound dehiscence. Overall, 84% to 89.5% of patients declared willingness to undergo further surgery in case of disease recurrence, and to recommend it to other patients, whereas about 9% would not choose the surgery again.

Wound Closure Techniques

It is believed that the relapse rate is primarily determined by the radicality of the excision and not by the wound closure technique.[3,7] Conversely, the relapse rate after primary closure was found to be much higher (54%) than the rates of split-thickness skin grafting (13%) or local flaps (19%).[50,51] In SIH, the relapse rate is low.[25,52] SIH is preferred by patients over skin grafting because of shorter hospital stay and sick leave, less limitation of mobility after surgery, and better cosmetic results.[25,53]

Other Factors Influencing the Risk of Relapse

Women are at greater risk of relapses than men.[8] Also, the location of HS influences the relapse rates. Inguinal, genital, and submammary HS relapse more frequently than axillary and perianal HS.[49,52]

SUMMARY

Surgical treatment in HS should be carried out by dermatosurgeons who have thorough knowledge of the pathology of the disease and excellent surgical skills. At least in more severe stages of HS, surgery should be introduced early after setting the diagnosis. Because the great impairment of quality of life in HS, patients are often highly motivated to change their condition by means of surgery. Preoperatively, medical treatment to calm active inflammation and imaging must be considered. Depending on the extent and severity of the disease local, tumescent, spinal, and/or general anesthesia are used. Incision and drainage can relieve pain in a setting of a tense, acute abscess. Deroofing is the primary surgical therapy for Hurley stage I/II. Until recently, wide excision was regarded as the preferred surgical method for Hurley stage II/III. The STEEP procedure seems to be a promising alternative to wide excision because it saves healthy tissue to a maximum and achieves complete removal of lesional tissue. After wide excision, different wound closure techniques can be chosen. Simple sutures can be used in small defects surrounded by loose skin. Split-thickness skin grafts are used typically for large wounds. Especially in genital and inguinal areas, flaps can be used successfully. However, the use of flap reconstruction, which is definitive by its nature, may not be appropriate in this disease with significant risk of progression. SIH ensures usually good functional and cosmetic results in defects of up to 140 cm^2. By using different techniques simultaneously, the benefits of the individual techniques can be combined.

REFERENCES

1. Revuz J, Jemec G. Diagnosing hidradentis suppurativa. Derm Clin, in press.

2. Weyandt G. Operative therapie der acne inversa. Hautarzt 2005;56:1033–9.
3. Rompel R, Petres J. Long-term results of wide surgical excision in 106 patients with hidradenitis suppurativa. Dermatol Surg 2000;26(7):638–43.
4. Wolkenstein P, Loundou A, Barrau K, et al, Quality of Life Group of the French Society of Dermatology. Quality of life impairment in hidradenitis suppurativa: a study of 61 cases. J Am Acad Dermatol 2007; 56(4):621–3.
5. Deckers IE, Kimball AB. The handicap of hidradentis suppurativa. Derm Clin, in press.
6. van der Zee HH, Prens EP, Boer J. Deroofing: a tissue-saving surgical technique for the treatment of mild to moderate hidradenitis suppurativa lesions. J Am Acad Dermatol 2010;63(3):475–80.
7. Kagan RJ, Yakuboff KP, Warner P, et al. Surgical treatment of hidradenitis suppurativa: a 10-year experience. Surgery 2005;138(4):734–40 [discussion: 740–1].
8. Blok JL, Boersma M, Terra JB, et al. Surgery under general anaesthesia in severe hidradenitis suppurativa: a study of 363 primary operations in 113 patients. J Eur Acad Dermatol Venereol 2015;29(8):1590–7.
9. Wortsman X. Imaging of hidradenitis suppurativa. Derm Clin, in press.
10. Zarchi K, Yazdanyar N, Yazdanyar S, et al. Pain and inflammation in hidradenitis suppurativa correspond to morphological changes identified by high-frequency ultrasound. J Eur Acad Dermatol Venereol 2015;29(3):527–32.
11. Church JM, Fazio VW, Lavery IC, et al. The differential diagnosis and comorbidity of hidradenitis suppurativa and perianal Crohn's disease. Int J Colorectal Dis 1993;8(3):117–9.
12. Klein JA. Anesthetic formulation of tumescent solutions. Dermatol Clin 1999;17(4):751–9, v–vi.
13. Glowacka K, Orzechowska-Juzwenko K, Bieniek A, et al. Optimization of lidocaine application in tumescent local anesthesia. Pharmacol Rep 2009;61(4): 641–53.
14. Namias A, Kaplan B. Tumescent anesthesia for dermatologic surgery. Cosmetic and noncosmetic procedures. Dermatol Surg 1998;24(7):755–8.
15. Ellis LZ. Hidradenitis suppurativa: surgical and other management techniques. Dermatol Surg 2012; 38(4):517–36.
16. Mullins JF, Mccash WB, Boudreau RF. Treatment of chronic hidradenitis suppurativa: surgical modification. Postgrad Med 1959;26:805–8.
17. Brown SC, Kazzazi N, Lord PH. Surgical treatment of perineal hidradenitis suppurativa with special reference to recognition of the perianal form. Br J Surg 1986;73(12):978–80.
18. Culp CE. Chronic hidradenitis suppurativa of the anal canal. A surgical skin disease. Dis Colon Rectum 1983;26(10):669–76.
19. van Hattem S, Spoo JR, Horvath B, et al. Surgical treatment of sinuses by deroofing in hidradenitis suppurativa. Dermatol Surg 2012;38(3):494–7.
20. Blok JL, Spoo JR, Leeman FW, et al. Skin-tissue-sparing excision with electrosurgical peeling (STEEP): a surgical treatment option for severe hidradenitis suppurativa Hurley stage II/III. J Eur Acad Dermatol Venereol 2015;29(2):379–82.
21. Greeley PW. Plastic surgical treatment of chronic suppurative hidradenitis. Plast Reconstr Surg (1946) 1951;7(2):143–6.
22. Stein A, Sebastian G. Acne inversa. Hautarzt 2003; 54(2):173–85 [quiz: 186–7].
23. Pollock WJ, Virnelli FR, Ryan RF. Axillary hidradenitis suppurativa. A simple and effective surgical technique. Plast Reconstr Surg 1972;49(1):22–7.
24. Ramasastry SS, Conklin WT, Granick MS, et al. Surgical management of massive perianal hidradenitis suppurativa. Ann Plast Surg 1985;15(3): 218–23.
25. Morgan WP, Harding KG, Hughes LE. A comparison of skin grafting and healing by granulation, following axillary excision for hidradenitis suppurativa. Ann R Coll Surg Engl 1983;65(4):235–6.
26. Morgan WP, Harding KG, Richardson G, et al. The use of silastic foam dressing in the treatment of advanced hidradenitis suppurativa. Br J Surg 1980;67(4):277–80.
27. Greenbaum AR. Modified abdominoplasty as a functional reconstruction for recurrent hydradenitis suppurativa of the lower abdomen and groin. Plast Reconstr Surg 2007;119(2):764–6.
28. Bieniek A, Matusiak L, Okulewicz-Gojlik D, et al. Surgical treatment of hidradenitis suppurativa: experiences and recommendations. Dermatol Surg 2010; 36(12):1998–2004.
29. Rieger UM, Erba P, Pierer G, et al. Hidradenitis suppurativa of the groin treated by radical excision and defect closure by medial thigh lift: aesthetic surgery meets reconstructive surgery. J Plast Reconstr Aesthet Surg 2009;62(10):1355–60.
30. Hudson D, Krige S. Axillary hidradenitis suppurativa – wide excision and flap coverage is best. Eur J Plast Surg 1993;16:94–7.
31. Geh JL, Niranjan NS. Perforator-based fasciocutaneous island flaps for the reconstruction of axillary defects following excision of hidradenitis suppurativa. Br J Plast Surg 2002;55(2):124–8.
32. Chuang CJ, Lee CH, Chen TM, et al. Use of a versatile transpositional flap in the surgical treatment of axillary hidradenitis suppurativa. J Formos Med Assoc 2004;103(8):644–7.
33. Schwabegger AH, Herczeg E, Piza H. The lateral thoracic fasciocutaneous island flap for treatment of recurrent hidradenitis axillaris suppurativa and other axillary skin defects. Br J Plast Surg 2000; 53(8):676–8.

34. Varkarakis G, Daniels J, Coker K, et al. Treatment of axillary hidradenitis with transposition flaps: a 6-year experience. Ann Plast Surg 2010;64(5):592–4.
35. Rehman N, Kannan RY, Hassan S, et al. Thoracodorsal artery perforator (TAP) type I V-Y advancement flap in axillary hidradenitis suppurativa. Br J Plast Surg 2005;58(4):441–4.
36. Blanc D, Tropet Y, Balmat P. Surgical treatment of suppurative axillary hidradenitis: value of a musculocutaneous island flap of the latissimus dorsi. Apropos of 3 cases. Ann Dermatol Venereol 1990;117(4):277–81.
37. Alharbi Z, Kauczok J, Pallua N. A review of wide surgical excision of hidradenitis suppurativa. BMC Dermatol 2012;12:9.
38. Rees L, Moses M, Clibbon J. The anterolateral thigh (ALT) flap in reconstruction following radical excision of groin and vulval hidradenitis suppurativa. J Plast Reconstr Aesthet Surg 2007;60(12):1363–5.
39. Solanki NS, Roshan A, Malata CM. Pedicled gracilis myocutaneous flap for treatment of recalcitrant hidradenitis suppurativa of the groin and perineum. J Wound Care 2009;18(3):111–2.
40. Kishi K, Nakajima H, Imanishi N. Reconstruction of skin defects after resection of severe gluteal hidradenitis suppurativa with fasciocutaneous flaps. J Plast Reconstr Aesthet Surg 2009;62(6):800–5.
41. Unal C, Yirmibesoglu OA, Ozdemir J, et al. Superior and inferior gluteal artery perforator flaps in reconstruction of gluteal and perianal/perineal hidradenitis suppurativa lesions. Microsurgery 2011;31(7):539–44.
42. Bieniek A, Matusiak L, Chlebicka I, et al. Secondary intention healing in skin surgery: our own experience and expanded indications in hidradenitis suppurativa, rhinophyma and non-melanoma skin cancers. J Eur Acad Dermatol Venereol 2013;27(8):1015–21.
43. Miller IM, Holtzman R, Hamzavi I. Prevalence, risk factors and co-morbidities of HS. Derm Clin, in press.
44. Lavogiez C, Delaporte E, Darras-Vercambre S, et al. Clinicopathological study of 13 cases of squamous cell carcinoma complicating hidradenitis suppurativa. Dermatology 2010;220(2):147–53.
45. Blackburn JH 2nd, Boemi L, Hall WW, et al. Negative-pressure dressings as a bolster for skin grafts. Ann Plast Surg 1998;40(5):453–7.
46. Elwood ET, Bolitho DG. Negative-pressure dressings in the treatment of hidradenitis suppurativa. Ann Plast Surg 2001;46(1):49–51.
47. Wormald JC, Balzano A, Clibbon JJ, et al. Surgical treatment of severe hidradenitis suppurativa of the axilla: thoracodorsal artery perforator (TDAP) flap versus split skin graft. J Plast Reconstr Aesthet Surg 2014;67(8):1118–24.
48. Boer J, Bos W, van der Meer B. Hidradenitis suppurativa (acne inversa): behandeling met deroofing en resorcine. Ned Tijdsch Derm & Ven 2004;14:274–8.
49. Ritz JP, Runkel N, Haier J, et al. Extent of surgery and recurrence rate of hidradenitis suppurativa. Int J Colorectal Dis 1998;13(4):164–8.
50. Watson JD. Hidradenitis suppurativa–a clinical review. Br J Plast Surg 1985;38(4):567–9.
51. Mandal A, Watson J. Experience with different treatment modules in hidradenitis suppuritiva: a study of 106 cases. Surgeon 2005;3(1):23–6.
52. Harrison BJ, Mudge M, Hughes LE. Recurrence after surgical treatment of hidradenitis suppurativa. Br Med J (Clin Res Ed) 1987;294(6570):487–9.
53. Meixner D, Schneider S, Krause M, et al. Acne inversa. J Dtsch Dermatol Ges 2008;6(3):189–96.

Lasers and Intense Pulsed Light Hidradenitis Suppurativa

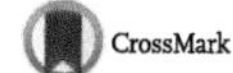

Ditte M. Saunte, MD, PhD[a,*], Jan Lapins, MD, DMSc[b]

KEYWORDS

• CO_2 laser • Laser • IPL • Carbon dioxide • Hidradenitis suppurativa • Intense pulsed light

KEY POINTS

- Lasers and intense pulsed light are useful in the treatment of hidradenitis suppurativa (HS).
- Carbon dioxide laser is used as a surgical instrument for cutting or vaporization of stationary HS elements.
- Hair removal by lasers and light devices destroys the hair follicles and thereby reduces the disease activity in the affected area.

INTRODUCTION: NATURE OF THE PROBLEM

The use of lasers and intense pulsed light (IPL) in the treatment of dermatologic conditions has increased over the past years. The carbon dioxide (CO_2) laser was the first used to treat hidradenitis suppurativa (HS) lesions. It is used as a surgical instrument for cutting or vaporization of the affected area with the advantage of a "blood-free" operation field and therefore removal with better control of subtle differences in the tissue. The better visualization provides the possibility of a macroscopic "Mohs-like" approach, in which only the minimum of tissue is removed.

More recently, other lasers and IPL targeting the hair have been tested and found useful.[1,2] The methods aim at reducing the numbers of hairs in areas with HS. In particular, the Nd:YAG laser is a promising therapeutic option because of its deep tissue penetration, but alexandrite laser, diode laser, and IPL have also been used in a limited number of studies. The studies all report improvement of HS after treatment.

CARBON DIOXIDE LASER

CO_2 laser vaporization surgery of HS was first introduced in 1987 by Sherman and Reid.[3] Initially, HS of the vulva was treated and later the method was extended for use in other body areas. In the early 1990s, with the arrival of scanners for CO_2 lasers, a smoother, faster, and safer removal of the pathologic tissues could be performed.

Treatment Goal and Planned Outcome

All operative techniques to treat HS aim at radically removing all keratinocytes and their potential remnants in nodules, abscesses, and tunnels. This can be done through excision en bloc of the whole involved skin area[4–6] or more selectively through vaporization of the pathologic tissue only[3,7–11] (**Table 1**).

Carbon dioxide laser excision surgery (en bloc)

CO_2 laser can be used to excise smaller or larger skin areas en bloc with or without laser coagulation of remnants (marsupialization) in the deep

Disclosures: D.M. Saunte was paid as a consultant for advisory board meeting by AbbVie and as a speaker for Bayer, Galderma, Astellas, and Leo Pharma. J. Lapins: nothing to declare.
[a] Department of Dermatology, Roskilde Hospital, Kogevej 7-13, Roskilde DK-4000, Denmark; [b] Department of Dermatology, Karolinska University Hospital, 171 76 Solna, Stockholm, Sweden
* Corresponding author.
E-mail address: disa@regionsjaelland.dk

Dermatol Clin 34 (2016) 111–119
http://dx.doi.org/10.1016/j.det.2015.08.001
0733-8635/16/$ – see front matter

Table 1
Carbon dioxide studies

Patients (Anatomic Sites)	Method	Anesthesia	Healing	Healing Time	Follow-up (Range)	Cure Rate[a]	Reference
Laser excision							
61 (185)	8–30 W	LA (99%)	SI	8.8 wk	1–19 y	98.9%	Hazen & Hazen,[5] 2010
9 (27)	18–40 W	GA (42%) LA (58%)	PC	NA 2–4 wk[b]	1 y	89.9%	Madan et al,[6] 2008
7 (13)	40 W	LA	SI	4–11 wk	10–27 mo	92%	Finley & Ratz,[4] 1996
Vaporization							
24	30 W, spot size 2 mm	LA	SI	3–5 wk	27 mo (15–47)	92%	Lapins et al,[7] 1994
34	Scanner-assisted, 20–30 W, spot size 3–6 mm	LA	SI	4–11 wk	34.5 mo (7–87)	88%	Lapins et al,[8] 2002
6	Narrow beam (1.6 mm), until depth 3–8 mm	NA	SI	3–7 wk	(9–36 mo)	100%	Dalrymple & Monaghan,[10] 1987
1	10–15 W	GA	Skin graft	NA	1 y	100%	Natarajan et al,[11] 2014
11	NA	NA	SI	2–8 wk	NA	100%	Sherman & Reid,[3] 1991
58	Scanner assisted 20–35 W, spot size 4 mm	GA LA	SI	NA	20.6 mo (1–47)	71%	Mikkelsen et al,[9] 2015

Abbreviations: CW, continuous wave; GA, general anesthesia; LA, local anesthesia; NA, not available.
[a] Cure rate of operation site.
[b] Went to work at week 2–4 postoperatively.

tissues, with less bleeding and better visualization than in standard excisions. This can also be achieved by electrosurgery, which may be used in a similarly tissue-sparing stepwise procedure.[12,13] This method is best suited for patients with stationary lesions (Hurley stages II-III). The reported results indicate a cure rate of 89.9% to 98.9% for specific lesions (see **Table 1**).[4–6]

Carbon dioxide laser vaporization surgery (selective focal treatment)

Scanner-assisted CO_2 laser treatment aims at focal radical treatment through vaporization of all nodules, abscesses, and fistulas, leaving healthy tissues in between the pathologic lesions untouched. This method is best suited for patients with smaller stationary lesions.

Starting in the center of a lesion, the tissue is vaporized in layers in a stepwise manner. The procedure is guided continuously by macroscopic inspection of the visible pathologic tissues and the goal is to remove all diseased tissue and reach healthy tissues in all directions, that is, complete removal both laterally and in depth. In this way, the technique can be tissue sparing and at the same time radical, much in analogy to the principles of Mohs surgery. Normal skin in between the HS lesions is left untouched and the wounds are left to healing by secondary intention. The reported cure rates are between 71% and 100% (see **Table 1**).[3,7–11]

Preoperative Planning and Preparation

The diseased skin is examined macroscopically for scarring, tissue distortion, and discoloration; dry or suppurating sinuses; macropseudocomedones; and other superficial signs. Symptomatic lesions are selected for the treatment (ie, those with discharge, inflammation, infiltration, or suspected abscesses). Areas that had been asymptomatic for more than 2 years but show signs of previous activity (eg, scars with postinflammatory hyperpigmentation, and sometimes with dry pseudocomedones) but no current inflammation are usually not treated. The examination is completed by palpating the defects for bulky indurations and small, firm subcutaneous nodules or fluctuating purulent tissue. The affected areas are delineated with ink.[14] Excised tissue en bloc or a preoperative biopsy for histopathology is recommended to exclude squamous cell carcinoma if clinically suspected.

Anesthesia

The choice of local or general anesthesia depends on the size and numbers of areas to be excised. Several approaches are outlined by Horvath and colleagues.[13]

Operative Techniques

In general, 2 different CO_2 laser methods are used: vaporization and excision (combined with marsupialization).

Vaporization technique

A scanner-assisted CO_2 laser is used. This is a laser with a focusing handpiece attached to the miniature optomechanical flash scanner delivery system that generates a focal spot, which moves rapidly and homogeneously in spiral scans and covers a round area on tissue at the focal plane. The area selected is gradually ablated by the laser beam when it passes over the tissue repeatedly. The aim of this procedure is to reduce thermal damage to adjacent tissue. Devitalized tissue is removed gently by cleansing the surface with swabs soaked in 0.9% sodium chloride solution. The depth of the vaporization is controlled by the selection of power, focal length, scanner-controlled spot size, and the movements of the handheld scanner. Often, 20 to 50 W, a spot size of 3 to 6 mm, and a focal length setting of 12.5 or 18 cm can be used. The vaporization procedure is repeated in downward and outward directions until fresh yellow adipose tissue is exposed in the deep, relatively thin, and anatomically normal skin margins laterally, with no remaining dense or discolored tissue. Usually, the vaporization reached the deep subcutaneous fat or fascia. In the axillary and inguinal regions, major vessels and the nerve plexus must be protected, but this depth is seldom reached in Hurley stage II lesions. The smaller blood vessels are coagulated by the laser, but bleeding from vessels larger than 0.5 to 1 mm in diameter is usually better addressed by electrocoagulation or ligation.[3,7–11] The use of scanner-assisted CO_2 laser surgery on a case of axillary hidradenitis suppurativa is shown in **Fig. 1**.

Excision technique

The diseased area is excised with the CO_2 laser using a small spot size (0.1–0.2 mm), continuous wave, and a high effect ($\leq$40 W).[4–6] In 2 studies, the laser was used in a defocused mode to vaporize the base and margins of the operation field (marsupialization) after the excision.[5,15]

Postprocedural Care

Primary closure

Few studies with a limited number of patients have reported primary closure after CO_2 laser surgery or skin grafting 10 days after laser excision.[6,11] In 1 of 9 patients, the sutures dehisced on the postoperative day 2 and in 2 of 9 patients scar contracture not restricting limb mobility was noted.[6] One year follow-up after skin grafting was without recurrence.[11]

Secondary Intention Healing

The wound is covered with ointment impregnated dressings or hydrofiber dressings and a covering bandage attached with surgical adhesive tape or gauze underwear. The dressings are initially left on for 2 or 3 days without changing to prevent early bleeding.[8] Thereafter, the wound is cleaned and rinsed with tap water, and the bandage is changed as often as necessary, sometimes daily, pending complete healing.

Other authors use foam dressings (Mepilex border, Mölnlycke, Sweden) and change the dressings once or twice daily.[9] Dressings with antibiotic ointment (bacitracin/polymyxin B or mupirocine) have been used in some studies.[5,6]

Rehabilitation and Recovery

Postoperative hospitalization is not necessary. HS patients are often used to dressings as adjuvant care of their lesions, and therefore often able to change dressings without professional help. The wounds are inspected after 1 to 2 weeks and at 6 weeks.[8] Many studies report that the postoperative discomfort was less or equal to the pain related to the HS.[3,6,10] In 1 study by Lapins and colleagues,[8] 56% of the patients experienced postoperative pain that did interfere with their daily activities, but all patients were able to resume their job before 3 weeks. Oral ibuprofen in combination with paracetamol has been used for pain management, as well as other nonsteroidal antiinflmmatory drugs such as ketorolac intramuscularly (intraoperative) and orally (postoperative).[4,9]

Postprocedural Course

Reepithelialization depends on the area evaporated, but is usually complete within 6 weeks

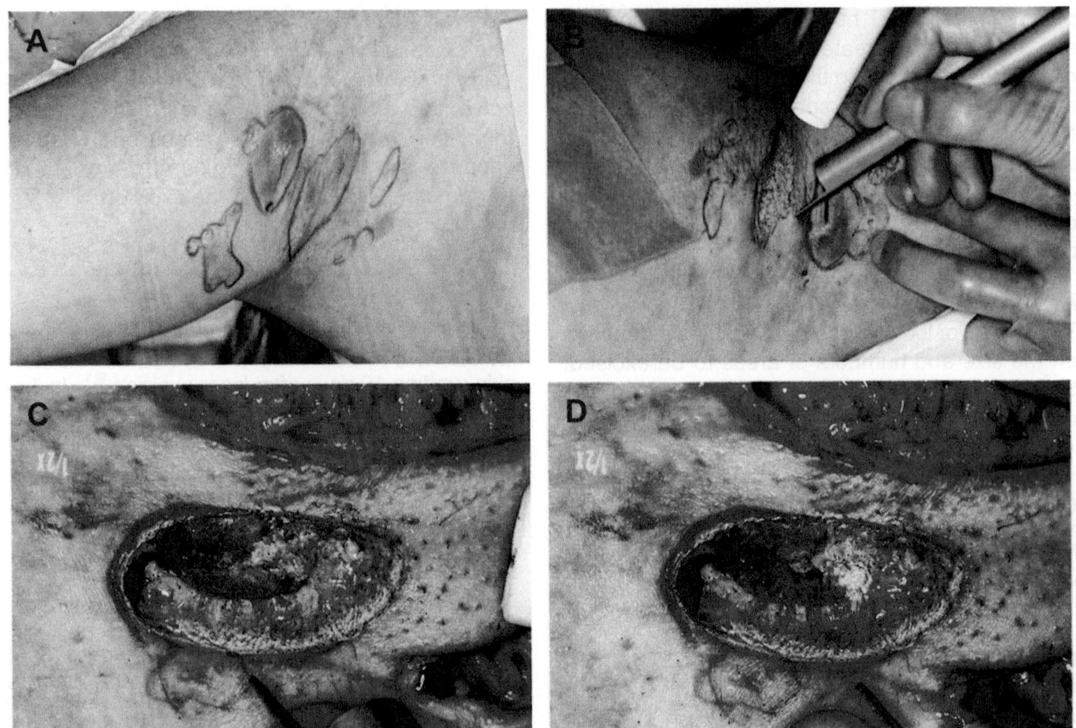

Fig. 1. A 42-year-old woman. Lesions have been delineated in ink after anesthesia before (*A*) and during (*B*) scanner assisted carbon dioxide laser surgery on hidradenitis suppurativa lesions of axilla with (*C*) and (*D*) close ups, respectively. (*From* Lapins J, Sartorius K, Emtestam L. Scanner-assisted carbon dioxide laser surgery: a retrospective follow-up study of patients with hidradenitis suppurativa. J Am Acad Dermatol 2002;47(2):281; with permission.)

(range, 2–11) for both CO_2 vaporization and the excision technique.[3–11] A case of secondary healing after CO_2 vaporization surgery is shown in **Fig. 2**. No studies have, however, compared the wound size with the healing time.

The most common complication is hypergranulation, infection (cellulitis), recurrence in the margin of the surgical area, scar contracture (axillary), and very rarely temporary paresthesia of the arm after axillary surgery.[3–11] One study identified obesity as a risk factor for recurrence.[9]

Clinical Results in the Literature

Results of clinical studies of CO_2 lasers for excision and vaporization in HS are shown in **Table 1**. The CO_2 laser has also been used to treat the HS scarring (fractionated CO_2) and to deroof sinus tracts in combination with hair removal.[16,17]

Summary

With good selection of patients, CO_2 laser is an efficient treatment of HS. In particular, patients with clearly separated, multiple, well-defined lesions are suitable. The advantages of the method are good vascular control, perioperative visibility of pathologic tissues, and sparing of healthy tissues. The technique is suitable for outpatient therapy. When the wound is healed by secondary intention, the risk of postoperative scar contractures is low.[6]

LASERS AND INTENSE PULSED LIGHT USED FOR HAIR REMOVAL IN THE TREATMENT OF HIDRADENITIS SUPPURATIVA

Since 1996, lasers and IPL have been used for hair removal mostly for cosmetic reasons.[18] However, in dermatology hair removal has also been used for the treatment of diseases, such as hirsutism, hypertricosis, and for hair-bearing skin grafts.

Based on the assumption that HS develops in the hair follicle, laser and IPL targeting the hair have been applied in the treatment of HS lesions (**Table 2**).[14] Overall, the number of studies and patients are few. In this section, different lasers and light studies applied in HS patients are reviewed.

Treatment Goal and Planned Outcome

Histologic studies have suggested that HS is a disorder of the terminal follicular epithelium with

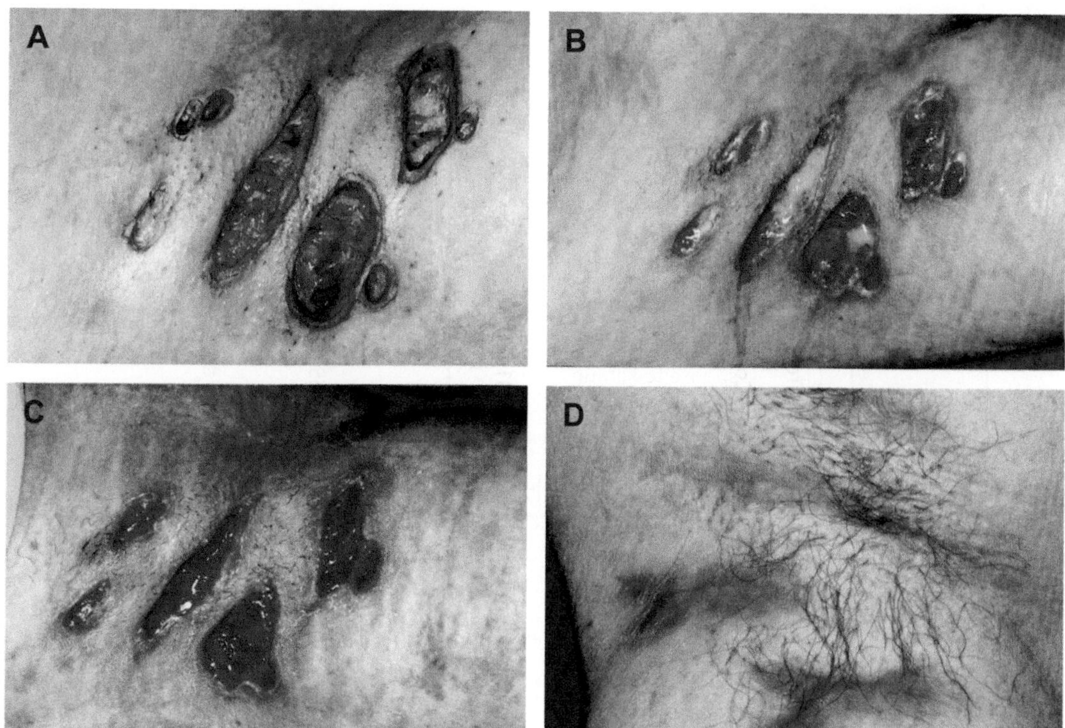

Fig. 2. Same woman as in Fig. 1. (A) Immediately after scanner-assisted carbon dioxide laser surgery performed on the axilla. (B) 1 One week. (C) Three weeks. (D) Three months later, healing by secondary intention. (*From* Lapins J, Sartorius K, Emtestam L. Scanner-assisted carbon dioxide laser surgery: a retrospective follow-up study of patients with hidradenitis suppurativa. J Am Acad Dermatol 2002;47(2):283; with permission.)

follicular hyperkeratosis and obstruction acting as an early event in the pathogenesis of HS.[19,20] The treatment goal for the hair removal lasers and light devices is, therefore, to destroy the hair follicles and thereby reduce the disease activity.

Nd:YAG Laser

The 1064-nm Nd:YAG laser can be used for depilation, and has been used in Hurley stage II and III in 3 prospective, randomized, controlled clinical trials with a total of 63 patients (see **Table 2**).[20–22] The Nd:YAG laser was used monthly for 2 to 4 months. The studies used a left–right comparative design with 1 side randomised for active Nd:YAG treatment and the contralateral site serving as the control.[20–22] In 2 studies,[20,22] the laser treatment was combined with bilateral use of topical benzoyl peroxide and clindamycin treatment. The effect was evaluated clinically (Sartorius score)[20–22] and by histology.[20,21] In all 3 studies, a significant decrease in Sartorius score (modified) from the baseline over all anatomic sites was found with a percent change improvement between 31.6% and 72%.[20–22] During treatment, either ultrasound gel and a cooling tip[20,22] or topical cooling gel, ice packs, and metal-tipped cooling device[21] were used for analgesia. Adverse effects reported were initial worsening of inflammation, which resolved within 1 week,[22] or transient pain.[20]

Long-pulsed 755-nm Alexandrite Laser (Cynosure Elite)

Only 1 case report has been published using alexandrite laser to the treatment of HS (see **Table 2**). The patient had Hurley stage II. Lidocaine/prilocaine mixture and an eutectic mixture of local anesthetics cream was used for anesthesia. No adverse effects were reported and the response was “excellent” at the 10-month follow-up.[23]

Diode Laser (1450 nm)

One case of axillary HS treated with diode laser (1450 nm) has been published (see **Table 2**).[24] Cryogen cooling spray and 4% tetracaine gel were used as anesthesia, but the patient nevertheless experienced pain during treatment. Partial improvement was achieved after 4 treatments and sweating was reduced notably.

Table 2
Laser systems and IPL used for treating HS by targeting the hair

Device	Patients (N)	Hurley Stage	Study Design	Settings	Controls	Method	Results	Reference
Laser								
1064-nm Nd:YAG long-pulsed	22	II	Prospective, controlled clinical (and histologic) study	Skin type I-III: Fluence: 40–50 J/cm^2 Spot size: 10 Pulse duration: 20 Skin type IV-VI: Fluence: 25–35 J/cm^2 Spot size: 10 mm Pulse duration: 35 ms	Treated area: Nd:YAG and topical treatment[b] Control area: contralateral site[b]	Monthly Nd:YAG for 4 mo	Treated: 72.7% improvement Controls: 22.9% improvement [a]	Mahmoud et al,[20] 2010
1064-nm Nd:YAG long-pulsed	19	II	Prospective, controlled clinical (and histologic) study	Skin type I-III: 40–50 J/cm^2, 20 ms, 10 mm spot Skin type IV-VI: 25–35 J/cm^2, 35 ms, 10 mm spot	Other anatomic site served as control	Two monthly laser sessions	31.6% improvement[a]	Xu et al,[21] 2011
1064-nm Nd:YAG long-pulsed	22	II/III	Prospective, randomized, controlled study	Skin type I-III: Fluence: 40–50 J/cm^2, Pulse duration: 20 ms Spot size: 10 mm Skin type IV-VI: Fluence: 25–35/Jcm^2 Pulse duration: 35 ms Spot size: 10 mm	Treated: Nd:YAG and topical treatment[b] Controls: topical treatment[b]	Three monthly laser sessions	65.3% improvement[a]	Tierney et al,[22] 2009

Alexandrite laser (long-pulsed 755-nm)	1	III	Retrospective review	Fluence 15–22 J/cm² Spot size: 15 Pulse duration 20 ms	No	6 treatments, 6- to 8-wk intervals	Improvement	Koch et al,[23] 2015
Diode laser (1450 nm)	1	NA	Case	Fluence 14 J/cm² Spot size: 6 mm DCD: 50 ms	No	4 treatments, intervals NA	Partial improvement	Downs,[24] 2004
Light								
IPL (filter 550)	2	I/II	Case	Hair removal: Fluence 7–9 J/cm², pulses 2–3, pulse duration 5 ms delay 10–20 ms Inflammatory components: Fluence 8–10 J/cm², pulses 2, pulse duration 5–10 ms delay 10 ms	No	4 sessions (hair mode) with 15–20 d interval and additional 2 sessions (inflammatory mode)	Improved (cured)	Piccolo et al,[25] 2014
IPL (420 nm)	18	II/III	Prospective study	Fluence 7–10 J/cm² Pulse duration: 30–50 ms	Contralateral side served as control	IPL twice per week for 4 wk	Improvement at months 12[a]	Highton et al,[26] 2011

Abbreviations: IPL, intense pulsed light; NA, Not available.

[a] Significant.

[b] Benzoyl peroxide and clindamycin.

Intense Pulsed Light

IPL is a polychromatic, noncoherent, and broad-spectrum pulsed light source (xenon lamp), which is able to emit light of a wavelength between 390 and 1200 nm.[25] The wavelength used in HS studies was 420 and 550 nm.[25,26] These wavelengths target melanin. It can therefore be used to destroy pigmented hairs by selective photothermolysis.[25]

Outcomes

IPL has been used in 1 prospective, randomized, patient-controlled clinical trial[26] including 18 patient with Hurley stages II to III (see **Table 2**). There was no information regarding use of anesthesia. The only reported adverse effect was erythema. A significant improvement was maintained 12 months after the treatment.[26] IPL has also been reported in 2 cases[25] with Hurley stages I and II (see **Table 2**). The IPL treatment resulted in complete removal of both inflammatory and painful components; hair removal was also achieved.[25]

Rehabilitation and recovery

Neither hospitalization nor sick leave is necessary after these procedures.

Summary

Removal of hair with lasers and light improves the HS symptoms in several studies, but repeated treatments seem to be necessary. Long-term follow-up is lacking.

OVERALL SUMMARY

Invasive CO_2 laser surgery as well as noninvasive hair removal by laser or IPL are local treatments with few (if any) systemic side effects. CO_2 laser surgery is an effective therapy for the removal of affected tissue in severe and recalcitrant HS with persistent sinus tract and scarring, and it can be performed under simple local infiltrative anesthesia. CO_2 laser does not prevent the development of new lesions, which, however, is one of the goals for hair removal methods. Hair removal by lasers and IPL improves the HS symptoms; however, the effect is temporary and need to be repeated. There is usually no downtime for recovery after treatment. CO_2 laser excision and vaporization as well as hair removal by laser and IPL are valuable methods to treat HS.

ACKNOWLEDGMENTS

The authors thank Professor Jemec for valuable comments and linguistic suggestions.

REFERENCES

1. Jemec GB, Hansen U. Histology of hidradenitis suppurativa. J Am Acad Dermatol 1996;34(6):994–9. Available at: www.ncbi.nlm.nih.gov/pubmed/8647993. Accessed March 25, 2015.
2. Yu CC, Cook MG. Hidradenitis suppurativa: a disease of follicular epithelium, rather than apocrine glands. Br J Dermatol 1990;122(6):763–9. Available at: www.ncbi.nlm.nih.gov/pubmed/2369556. Accessed March 25, 2015.
3. Sherman AI, Reid R. CO_2 laser for suppurative hidradenitis of the vulva. J Reprod Med 1991;36(2):113–7. Available at: www.ncbi.nlm.nih.gov/pubmed/2010892. Accessed March 10, 2015.
4. Finley EM, Ratz JL. Treatment of hidradenitis suppurativa with carbon dioxide laser excision and second-intention healing. J Am Acad Dermatol 1996;34(3):465–9. Available at: www.ncbi.nlm.nih.gov/pubmed/8609261. Accessed March 10, 2015.
5. Hazen PG, Hazen BP. Hidradenitis suppurativa: successful treatment using carbon dioxide laser excision and marsupialization. Dermatol Surg 2010;36(2):208–13.
6. Madan V, Hindle E, Hussain W, et al. Outcomes of treatment of nine cases of recalcitrant severe hidradenitis suppurativa with carbon dioxide laser. Br J Dermatol 2008;159(6):1309–14.
7. Lapins J, Marcusson JA, Emtestam L. Surgical treatment of chronic hidradenitis suppurativa: CO_2 laser stripping-secondary intention technique. Br J Dermatol 1994;131(4):551–6. Available at: www.ncbi.nlm.nih.gov/pubmed/7947209. Accessed March 10, 2015.
8. Lapins J, Sartorius K, Emtestam L. Scanner-assisted carbon dioxide laser surgery: a retrospective follow-up study of patients with hidradenitis suppurativa. J Am Acad Dermatol 2002;47(2):280–5. Available at: www.ncbi.nlm.nih.gov/pubmed/12140476. Accessed March 10, 2015.
9. Mikkelsen PR, Dufour DN, Zarchi K, et al. Recurrence rate and patient satisfaction of CO_2 laser evaporation of lesions in patients with hidradenitis suppurativa: a retrospective study. Dermatol Surg 2015;41(2):255–60.
10. Dalrymple JC, Monaghan JM. Treatment of hidradenitis suppurativa with the carbon dioxide laser. Br J Surg 1987;74(5):420. Available at: www.ncbi.nlm.nih.gov/pubmed/3109537. Accessed March 10, 2015.
11. Natarajan K, Srinivas CR, Thomas M, et al. Hidradenitis suppurativa treated with carbon dioxide laser followed by split skin thickness graft. Indian J Dermatol Venereol Leprol 2014;80(4):376–8.
12. Blok JL, Spoo JR, Leeman FWJ, et al. Skin-tissue-sparing excision with electrosurgical peeling (STEEP): a surgical treatment option for severe

hidradenitis suppurativa Hurley stage II/III. J Eur Acad Dermatol Venereol 2015;29(2):379–82.

13. Janse I, Bieniek A, Horváth B, et al. Surgical procedures in hidradenitis suppurativa. Dermatol Clin, in press

14. Zouboulis CC, Desai N, Emtestam L, et al. European S1 guideline for the treatment of hidradenitis suppurativa/acne inversa. J Eur Acad Dermatol Venereol 2015;29(4):619–44.

15. Hazen PG, Daoud S. Scrotal hidradenitis suppurativa with secondary lymphedema and lymphangiomata: successful management with carbon dioxide laser excision and marsupialization. Dermatol Surg 2015;41(3):431–2.

16. Krakowski AC, Admani S, Uebelhoer NS, et al. Residual scarring from hidradenitis suppurativa: fractionated CO_2 laser as a novel and noninvasive approach. Pediatrics 2014;133(1):e248–51.

17. Jain V, Jain A. Use of lasers for the management of refractory cases of hidradenitis suppurativa and pilonidal sinus. J Cutan Aesthet Surg 2012; 5(3):190–2.

18. Grossman MC, Dierickx C, Farinelli W, et al. Damage to hair follicles by normal-mode ruby laser pulses. J Am Acad Dermatol 1996;35(6):889–94. Available at: www.ncbi.nlm.nih.gov/pubmed/8959946. Accessed March 29, 2015.

19. Sellheyer K, Krahl D. "Hidradenitis suppurativa" is acne inversa! An appeal to (finally) abandon a misnomer. Int J Dermatol 2005;44(7):535–40.

20. Mahmoud BH, Tierney E, Hexsel CL, et al. Prospective controlled clinical and histopathologic study of hidradenitis suppurativa treated with the long-pulsed neodymium:yttrium-aluminium-garnet laser. J Am Acad Dermatol 2010;62(4):637–45.

21. Xu LY, Wright DR, Mahmoud BH, et al. Histopathologic study of hidradenitis suppurativa following long-pulsed 1064-nm Nd:YAG laser treatment. Arch Dermatol 2011;147(1):21–8.

22. Tierney E, Mahmoud BH, Hexsel C, et al. Randomized control trial for the treatment of hidradenitis suppurativa with a neodymium-doped yttrium aluminium garnet laser. Dermatol Surg 2009;35(8): 1188–98.

23. Koch D, Pratsou P, Szczecinska W, et al. The diverse application of laser hair removal therapy: a tertiary laser unit's experience with less common indications and a literature overview. Lasers Med Sci 2015; 30(1):453–67.

24. Downs A. Smoothbeam laser treatment may help improve hidradenitis suppurativa but not Hailey-Hailey disease. J Cosmet Laser Ther 2004;6:163–4. Available at: www.ncbi.nlm.nih.gov/pubmed/15545102. Accessed March 10, 2015.

25. Piccolo D, Di Marcantonio D, Crisman G, et al. Unconventional use of intense pulsed light. Biomed Res Int 2014;2014:618206.

26. Highton L, Chan W-Y, Khwaja N, et al. Treatment of hidradenitis suppurativa with intense pulsed light: a prospective study. Plast Reconstr Surg 2011; 128(2):459–65.

Index

Note: Page numbers of article titles are in **boldface** type.

Dermatol Clin 34 (2016) 121–128
http://dx.doi.org/10.1016/S0733-8635(15)00136-9
0733-8635/16/$ – see front matter

H

W

Z

Printed and bound by CPI Group (UK) Ltd, Croydon, CR0 4YY
03/10/2024
01040376-0013